MEDICARE
Demystified

A Physician Helps Save You
Time, Money, and Frustration

Ronald Kahan, MD

ISBN: 1495920461
ISBN 13: 9781495920462
Library of Congress Control Number: 2014902954
CreateSpace Independent Publishing Platform
North Charleston, South Carolina

To Betsy

Acknowledgements

I am indebted to those professionals who shared their areas of expertise with me.

- Sharon Bradley RN, Christine Pfeffer RN, and Mary Ross RN of Visiting Nurse and Hospice of Fairfield County

- Joe Pajor, Christine Pasiakos RN, and Joanne Svogun RN of Norwalk Hospital

- Richard Huntley MD, Michael Marks MD, Jason Orlinick MD, James Slater MD, and Stephen Winter MD

- Kathy Pajor RN and her staff at Beachwood Rehab and Nursing Center

- Kris Bokon of Kay and Co.

Friends and colleagues Bob Clay, Sue Cruikshank EdD, Michael Fenster MD, Jack Lapolla EdD and Fred Smith read and criticized the manuscript.

Particular thanks to Peter and Jackie Flatow whose ongoing advice and encouragement have been invaluable.

My editor, Christine Benton, showed me the right way to write a book.

Contents

Introduction

Denise Hoffman and Joann Green were having coffee one morning. They'd been friends since childhood and were lucky enough to have lived near each other all their lives. Joann had recently lost her husband of 38 years.

"You know, Denise, I'm still having such a hard time without Jim. I miss him terribly. He was always there for me and did so many things I just took for granted. Now I'm having to make decisions that I never even thought about before. Like my health insurance.

We always had good insurance through Jim's jobs, but now I have to figure out what to do about Medicare. I've been getting all kinds of stuff in the mail, and I see ads on TV. They talk about Medicare supplements and plans that replace regular Medicare with less paperwork. I have to decide in the next two months. I really want to be able to stay with Dr. Goodman. It's all very confusing, and I don't know where to turn."

I was born in 1945. At that time, my father was a country doctor in rural Illinois. He was the only physician for miles around and had to do whatever was needed for his patients. He delivered babies, set fractures, did surgery, and treated diseases with the few medicines available at that time. My father was paid in cash...or even in chickens; sometimes he received payment at the time he saw the patient, or sometimes many months later when resources were available. The medical delivery system was far simpler then, and so was the payment system.

Medicare wasn't available at that time, and the whole idea of medical insurance was only in its infancy. In the early 1930s health insurance programs had slowly crept into existence, with Blue Shield (later BlueCross and Blue Shield) being the earliest nonprofit insurer. The Hill-Burton Act of 1946 provided government funds to build new hospitals and improve old ones, resulting in a nationwide increase in the availability of care. Along with becoming more accessible, medical care was evolving and improving—and becoming more expensive.

There were no government-funded medical plans until the 1960s. On July 30, 1965, President Lyndon Johnson signed legislation that established Medicare and Medicaid. He made former president Harry Truman the first Medicare recipient to recognize his leadership in advocating for government medical insurance programs. Medicare was born. By July 1, 1966, there were 19 million Medicare enrollees. The Center for Medicare and Medicaid Services was created to administer these two programs. I'll refer to it frequently and use its nickname, CMS, for convenience.

Medicare has changed significantly since its inception. Originally it served only individuals age 65 and older. Today, it also covers people of all ages with certain physical and mental disabilities, as well as those with end-stage renal disease (kidney failure with need for dialysis or a kidney transplant) and those with ALS (amyotrophic lateral sclerosis, also known as Lou Gehrig's Disease).

In 1997, an alternative to traditional Medicare was added. Known as Medicare Advantage, it allowed Medicare recipients to opt for insurance programs sold by private insurance carriers. Either choice provided good coverage for doctors and hospitals, but the cost of medications was becoming a progressively greater portion of overall medical expenses. As a result, a prescription drug benefit was added when, in December 2003, President George W. Bush signed the Medicare Modernization Act. Coverage for seniors now encompassed all components of health care.

The Medicare system we have today has resulted from these major pieces of legislation, as well as smaller modifications. Medicare has evolved as changes in medical technology have necessitated reconsideration of what is covered and how. Additionally, CMS has been exploring new models of medical care delivery in the hope of improving care and delivering it more cost-effectively. It is clear that the price tag for Medicare is expanding at an unsustainable pace. Greater and greater numbers of people are being covered by Medicare, both because the baby boomers are now reaching age 65 and because people are living longer. Additionally, modern medicine is becoming ever more complex and thus more expensive. The cost of Medicare is already a major political issue; it will become more so in the future.

For years I have counseled patients on making educated choices about their Medicare coverage and have routinely heard, "I didn't realize that," or "Nobody told me." There is clearly an information gap regarding Medicare, and I want to close that gap.

When I sat down to write this book, my main goal was to fully explain Medicare, including its component parts, its options, and its costs. Since Medicare is even more complicated than it appears, the subtleties of decision-making, deadlines, and penalties are critical to Medicare recipients.

However, as I discussed the need for informed decision making with friends and colleagues, they told me that simply explaining the workings of Medicare wasn't enough. Sure, one needs to make wise choices when selecting a medical insurance package. But what about dealing with the health care system *after* you've chosen your medical coverage?

- How do you use your insurance to best advantage?

- To what extent will being insured by Medicare affect your ability to access care?

- Will doctors be willing to see you?

- Will hospitals treat you differently?

- How will you deal with the paperwork?

Clearly, the information gap extends far beyond figuring out which Medicare options to choose. Understanding how to navigate the medical system is every bit as important.

Selecting an appropriate Medicare program will be covered in the first portion of this book. The second part will deal with how to function effectively within our present health care system as it relates to seniors with Medicare. I'll discuss how to select a doctor and barriers to finding one. I'll talk about going to the hospital and options for post-hospital care. I'll touch on some newer concepts such as concierge medicine and ponder the future of Medicare. And more.

What I won't discuss, however, is anything about specific diseases or treatments. This book is not a medical textbook. It's not designed to teach you about your body in health and disease. You'll find nothing about how to prevent, diagnose, or treat any medical condition. What you will understand, though, is how to use the health care system so it works for you. When you know the system, you'll make better choices for your health, your pocketbook, and your peace of mind.

THIS BOOK IS A MANUAL FOR SURVIVAL UNDER MEDICARE TODAY.

Part I

Choosing Your Medicare Plan

Chapter 1

The Basics of Medicare

"Happy Birthday to me. Happy Birthday to me. Happy Birthday, dear Bobbie. Happy Birthday to me. 65. Unbelievable. Free as a bird. Just one thing: The benefits people over at my old company said I had to sign up for Medicare or my retiree medical benefits wouldn't continue; and I'll have to pay some premiums. What's that all about? I guess I'll have to find out about Medicare. I'll do it tomorrow. Today, Happy Birthday to me!"

Who Qualifies for Medicare?

For seniors, two simple criteria must be met to qualify for Medicare:

1. You must be 65 years old.

2. You must be a U.S. citizen or a legal resident of the U.S. for five continuous years.

That's it. There are no additional requirements. It doesn't matter how long you have worked or how many years you have paid FICA (Social Security) or Medicare taxes.

If neither you nor your spouse has paid FICA taxes for at least 10 years, Medicare will cost you more, but you're still eligible for coverage.

All Medicare insurance policies are *individual* policies. Couples policies, family policies, and the like do not exist in Medicare. Additionally, the age of your spouse has no bearing on your Medicare eligibility. *You* must be 65; your spouse's age is irrelevant.

Medicare Before Age 65

There are ways to qualify for Medicare without reaching age 65. Individuals with certain physical or emotional disabilities, who have received Social Security disability benefits for two years, may then receive Medicare. Disability under Social Security is determined on a case-by-case basis. Patients with end-stage renal disease (kidney failure) who require dialysis or a kidney transplant also qualify, as do those with a disease called ALS (Lou Gehrig's disease).

Making Choices

Medicare is definitely not a single program. There are lots of options, and you'll have to make many choices as you go along. I'll try to guide you through the maze of options so you can make the best decisions for your particular needs.

Once you've decided it's time to enroll in Medicare, your first choice point involves picking one of the two basic forms of Medicare

1. **Original Medicare**

    OR

2. **Medicare Advantage**

Following is a simplified overview of the two options and their various components. Note that Chapters 2 through 6 will provide in-depth analyses of both.

OPTION #1: ORIGINAL MEDICARE

The term **Original Medicare** refers to Medicare as it has evolved since its inception in 1965. You may sometimes see references to "regular Medicare" or "traditional Medicare." They all mean the same thing, but the correct term is Original Medicare, and that's what I'll use in this book.

IF YOU HEAR THE TERM "REGULAR MEDICARE" OR "TRADITIONAL MEDICARE," IT MEANS WHAT IS OFFICIALLY KNOWN AS ORIGINAL MEDICARE.

Whether you've had medical insurance provided by an employer or you bought the plan yourself, it was more than likely a single program that covered doctors, hospitals, and drugs, and you probably had one insurance card. As you'll see, Original Medicare works very differently. A complete Original Medicare insurance package includes several component parts:

- **Medicare Part A (inpatient care)**

  Inpatient care (medical, surgical, psychiatric, or rehabilitative) including hospital stays, some care in skilled nursing facilities after hospitalization, hospice care, and some home health care.

  The Center for Medicare and Medicaid Services (CMS) administers Medicare Part A. It's *premium-free* for most people. However, recipients do have cost sharing responsibility through deductibles, coinsurance, and copays.

- **Medicare Part B (doctors and outpatient care)**

  Doctors' fees (primary care and specialists, both in and out of hospitals) and ambulatory care. Part B outpatient services are extensive and include ER and ambulance services; X-rays, scans, and laboratory tests; outpatient surgery; physical, occupational therapy; and preventive services. (A complete list of Part B outpatient services appears at the beginning of Chapter 3.)

  CMS also administers Part B. Recipients pay a monthly premium and cost sharing applies for most services.

- **Medicare Part D (prescription drug coverage)**

  Many prescription drugs but *no* over-the-counter ones. Part D plans are policies provided by private insurance companies under Medicare guidelines. Plans vary widely in cost and which drugs are included; individuals share the cost through varying combinations of monthly premiums, deductibles, and copays. (Chapter 5 contains detailed information about Part D—the most complicated part of Medicare.)

- **Medicare Supplement Insurance Policies (Medigap Policy)**

  Some individuals choose to take out an additional policy to cover the cost sharing inherent in Medicare Parts A and B. (Chapter 4 addresses Medigap options in detail.)

To have fairly complete coverage under Original Medicare, you would have three separate policies and three separate insurance cards:

- **a red, white, and blue Medicare Card for Parts A and B**

- **a Medicare Part D insurance card**

- **a Medicare Supplement card**

Cost Sharing Under Medicare

Both Original Medicare and Medicare Advantage plans require you to pay part of the cost of your care (although you can sometimes buy insurance to cover these costs). The amount you must pay can take several forms—deductibles, copayments, and coinsurance.

- **Deductible**—A deductible refers to the amount you must pay before the plan pays *anything*. A deductible is a specific dollar amount. It may be an annual deductible, which is an amount you must pay *each year* before the plan starts paying. Or it may refer to some other specific time period or event, such as a hospitalization. For example, Medicare Part A requires that you pay a deductible of $1,216 for a hospital admission; Medicare Part B requires a $147 deductible each year before the plan begins to pay.

- **Copayment** (more commonly called a **copay**)—A copay is a fixed dollar amount that you must pay each time you receive a service or product. For example, a Medicare Advantage plan might require a $10 copay when you see your family doctor, or a Medicare Drug Plan might charge a $6 copay for a generic prescription medication.

- **Coinsurance**—Unlike a deductible or copay, coinsurance is *not* a fixed dollar amount. Rather, it is a *percentage* of the total cost of a service or product. For example, under Medicare Part B, when you see a participating doctor you are responsible for coinsurance of 20% of the Medicare-approved fee. Similarly, a particular Medicare Advantage plan might require you to pay 30% coinsurance for consulting a physician outside the plan's approved provider list.

<u>Note:</u> The term **coinsurance** frequently causes confusion. Some people think coinsurance refers to additional medical insurance that covers some or all of what Original Medicare doesn't. The correct term for that type of insurance is **secondary insurance** or **supplemental insurance**. From Medicare's point of view, the term **coinsurance** refers specifically to the percentage of a fee that is *your* responsibility, not Medicare's.

"Helps to pay for..."—When you read materials put out by Medicare, whether in print or online, you will continually read the phrase "helps to pay for," referring to services that Medicare covers. Since Medicare coverage requires cost sharing (involving deductibles, copays, and coinsurance), it's not really correct to say that "Medicare pays for..." any given doctor's visit, hospitalization, or test, since Medicare is not paying the entire cost. That's why "helps to pay for" is used. I prefer to use the phrase "Medicare covers" to refer to any service that CMS considers part of Medicare's constellation of covered services, with the understanding that Medicare will often not be paying the total amount.

OPTION #2: MEDICARE ADVANTAGE (MEDICARE PART C)

As mentioned earlier, an alternative to Original Medicare exists: **Medicare Part C.** Known as Medicare Advantage (MA) plans and sometimes referred to as Medicare Health Plans, such programs are managed by private insurance companies but are subject to specific Medicare rules and regulations. CMS pays these plans a fixed dollar amount per month to provide all of an individual's care, but copays, deductibles, and coinsurance also apply.

A Medicare Advantage plan participant has *only* Medicare Part C— it replaces Medicare Part A and Part B and makes a Medigap policy unnecessary. Part D drug coverage is usually included as well.

Most Medicare Advantage plans use the concept of managed care, meaning you have a primary care doctor who coordinates your care and makes referrals for lab work, specialists, and procedures. This is different from Original Medicare, in which patients may see any doctor without a referral, as long as the physician accepts Medicare patients. In addition, Medicare Advantage programs generally rely on their own provider networks, and benefits often vary if patients choose doctors or medical facilities that are out-of-network.

According to data from the Henry J. Kaiser Family Foundation, about 72% of Medicare recipients are currently covered by Original Medicare, while 28% have opted for Medicare Advantage; and the percent enrolled in Medicare Advantage plans has more than doubled over the last ten years (from 13% in 2004). The appeal of Medicare Advantage is usually price, since a comprehensive medical insurance program can typically be obtained more reasonably with Medicare Advantage than with Original Medicare plus Medigap.

When and How Do I Sign Up?

When you turn 65, you're Medicare coverage can begin, but you should think about signing up well before that.

▶ *If you're already receiving Social Security retirement benefits:* Medicare will contact you several months before your 65th birthday. You will automatically be enrolled in Medicare Part A and Medicare Part B. You'll get a red, white, and blue Medicare card in the mail. Signing up for a Medicare Drug Plan (Medicare Part D) is not automatic, but you will get lots of information on how to do it. Similarly, you'll probably be inundated with solicitations encouraging you to buy various Medigap plans (and Medicare Advantage plans as well).

▶ *If you're not on Social Security:* You'll have to sign up yourself during what is called the **Initial Enrollment Period**—a seven-month period that includes:

- The three months immediately prior to your 65th birthday

- The month of your 65th birthday

- The three months immediately after your 65th birthday

⚠ **Be sure to sign up for Medicare during the Initial Enrollment Period, even if you're going to turn down some benefits, since you can pay significant penalties for waiting and signing up later.**

In some situations it may be advisable to defer starting certain parts of Medicare, particularly if you have other insurance. However, you'll almost certainly want to accept at least Part A coverage during the Initial Enrollment Period. I'll discuss this in detail later in Chapter 2.

Signing up yourself is easy. The simplest way is on the Internet at www.socialsecurity.gov (not at www.medicare.gov). If you're not comfortable with the Internet, or you have certain questions you want answered before you enroll, you can do so on the phone by calling Social Security at 1-800-772-1213. You will have to provide some information about yourself, including your Social Security number.

⚠ **It's important to understand the relationship between Medicare and Social Security and the difference between Medicare and Medicaid.**

The Relationship Between Medicare and Social Security

You should keep in mind that Medicare and Social Security are two separate programs. Certainly there are relationships between the two:

- How long you and your spouse have paid Social Security taxes determines whether you get free Medicare Part A.

- You sign up for Medicare through Social Security.

- If you are receiving Social Security payments, your monthly premiums for participating in Medicare can be deducted from your Social Security payments.

- Your Medicare card will use your Social Security number plus a letter as your Medicare ID.

- Many of your questions regarding Medicare can be answered at your local Social Security office.

But in terms of when you start receiving benefits, the two programs are *totally different:*

- You can begin receiving partial Social Security retirement benefits well before age 65, or you can defer your benefits until as late as age 70½. When you begin Medicare is unrelated to when you start receiving Social Security. For seniors, Medicare eligibility commences at age 65, period.

- You must enroll in Medicare at specified times, depending on your age and employment status, and there are penalties for not doing so. These requirements (and the resulting penalties) take effect even if you haven't started receiving Social Security payments.

Medicare Versus Medicaid

Medicare and Medicaid are also entirely different programs. Both come under the purview of the same organization—the Center for Medicare and Medicaid Services (CMS). However, the criteria for receiving the benefits of these two programs are quite disparate.

As noted, Medicare is for all seniors plus some individuals with disabilities and specific diseases. The vast majority of Medicare recipients are age 65 and older. Income level and how much money one has in the bank are irrelevant.

On the other hand, Medicaid provides medical services for the poor. It is funded jointly by federal and state governments. Eligibility for Medicaid, and therefore the number of people covered by the program, varies greatly from state to state. Much of Medicaid is oriented toward health care for children, pregnant women, and families with dependent children; however, some low-income adults and the disabled also qualify. The Affordable Care Act (ObamaCare) significantly increases the number of people who qualify for Medicaid.

Medicaid is heavily involved in paying for long-term custodial care in nursing homes, whereas Medicare provides no coverage whatever for custodial care. When an individual receives both Medicare and Medicaid benefits, Medicare is the primary insurance with Medicaid filling in the gaps.

When Will My Medicare Coverage Start?

▶ *If you enroll during the three month period prior to your 65th birthday:* Your coverage will begin the first day of the month of your 65th birthday.

▶ *If you sign up during the month of your birthday or any of the subsequent three months:* Your coverage will begin in the month after you sign up.

A special note for anyone whose birthday falls on the first day of the month: You get a better deal, since your coverage begins on the first day of the **previous** month, provided you've signed up prior to that month. I have no idea why.

Recommendation: Sign up as early in your Initial Enrollment Period as possible. First of all, why delay coverage? Medicare is a very good deal. If you are paying for your own insurance, Medicare will almost invariably be a more economical choice. Get it as soon as you can.

Remember that there are additional decisions you have to make regarding the other components of Medicare. You'll probably need a Part D (Medicare Drug Plan) policy and a Medicare Supplement (Medigap) policy. Alternatively, you may decide that having a Medicare Advantage plan (Medicare Part C) is a better choice for you. It takes time to make smart decisions. If you start studying your options early, you'll have a comprehensive insurance package ready to go as soon as you become eligible.

What if I Miss My Initial Enrollment Period?

If you don't sign up for Medicare during the Initial Enrollment Period, all is not lost. You won't lose your right to participate in Medicare. You can still enroll between January 1st and March 31st of any subsequent year during what's called a **General Enrollment Period.** Your coverage will then begin on July 1st of that year.

Be aware, however, that you won't be covered by Medicare while you're waiting for July 1st to roll around. If you have no other insurance, getting sick can be costly. Also, there are generally financial penalties for waiting. I'll discuss how these onerous penalties are assessed later on.

⚠ **Failure to sign up for Medicare during the Initial Enrollment Period can result in additional premiums for Medicare Parts B and D that continue indefinitely. Delays in starting Medicare Part A can also result in penalties for some people. Be very careful of this!**

Can I Delay Enrolling if I'm Still Working and Have Good Insurance?

Yes you can; and when you finally need Medicare, you'll be able to sign up during a **Special Enrollment Period** that's designed specifically for individuals who have continued to work past age 65 and their spouses. You are entitled to a Special Enrollment Period if you've been covered by a health plan provided by an employer, either your employer or your spouse's.

You may enroll in Medicare using the Special Enrollment Period provision any time *up to eight months after you cease to be covered by the employer-sponsored plan,* either because you (or your spouse) no longer works there or because the plan terminated.

To qualify you for a Special Enrollment Period, the employer's plan must be considered "creditable," which means that it provides coverage at least as good as Medicare does. The concept of "creditable coverage" will come up over and over again as I discuss various parts of Medicare.

Failing to sign up during the eight-month period means you'll have to wait for the next General Enrollment Period and be subject to penalties.

⚠ **Special Enrollment Periods do NOT apply to retiree insurance plans or COBRA.**

⚠ **Beware: Delaying enrollment in Medicare because you're covered by a retiree plan will NOT prevent you from incurring stiff penalties when you do finally enroll in Medicare.**

In summary, there are three different times you can sign up:

1. During the **Initial Enrollment Period,** which is the seven-month period that includes the three months before your 65th birthday, the month of your birthday, and the three months after your birthday.

2. During any subsequent **General Enrollment Period** (January 1st through March 31st), with coverage beginning on July 1st of that year.

3. During a **Special Enrollment Period,** which lasts for eight months after coverage under an employer-sponsored health plan ends. This is for individuals who have continued to work past age 65 and their spouses.

How Do I Communicate with Medicare?

It's easy to contact Medicare, both for general information and to get your specific questions answered. CMS provides some useful informational tools.

- There are brochures and pamphlets, the most comprehensive of which is called *Medicare and You*. It comes out yearly and, as it says on the cover, "This is the official U.S. Government Medicare Handbook." It's available free from CMS. You should receive one automatically; if not, you can request one. The copy you receive in the mail will include some information specific to your locality, which can be very useful.

- There is also a wealth of information on the Medicare website, www.medicare.gov. It covers the same material found in *Medicare and You* plus much, much more. Also, it includes some helpful interactive tools that are indispensable when comparing plans.

  For example, in evaluating Medicare Part D drug plans, you can use an online program called the *Medicare Plan Finder*. You plug in the drugs you presently take and it will tell you how your medications would be covered under different plans you may be considering. When appropriate, I will make specific references to Medicare web addresses that provide pertinent information or useful tools.

⚠ **Make sure to use the suffix *.gov* for the Internet addresses of all Medicare and CMS websites. *Never* use *.com* or *.net.* For example, www. Medicare.com is NOT an official Medicare website.**

- You also can call Medicare at 1-800-MEDICARE to ask general questions or ones that apply specifically to you. The representatives are very helpful. If there are long waits, the automated system will ask you to provide a telephone number where you can be reached so you won't have to wait on hold. They really do call you back!

  For some services, you may be asked to make a telephone appointment with someone who can help you with your particular problem. You will be called very close to your scheduled time.

- Another excellent source of individualized Medicare information and counseling is your State Health Insurance Assistance Program (SHIP). The telephone number of your particular state's SHIP office can be found on the back cover of the *Medicare and You* copy you receive in the mail; alternatively, you can find it at www.medicare.gov or by calling 1-800-MEDICARE.

Chapter 2

Medicare Part A

"Did you say that Medicare Part A was free? Really? Free? Awesome!"

What Does Medicare Part A Cover?

Medicare Part A covers *inpatient* care, whether medical, surgical, psychiatric, or rehabilitative. This includes hospital stays as well as some care in skilled nursing facilities after a hospitalization, hospice care, and some home health care. It does NOT cover doctors' fees, even in a hospital—they're covered by Medicare Part B. But let's be more specific:

HOSPITAL ADMISSION

If you're admitted to a hospital for a "medically necessary" reason, Medicare Part A will cover the following services:

- A semiprivate room (or private room if deemed medically necessary)

- Meals

- Skilled nursing care

- Operating and recovery rooms

- Intensive care and coronary care units

- Laboratory tests

- X-ray tests and scans, including specialized ones like CT scans and MRIs

- Medications given in the hospital

- Medical equipment and supplies used in the hospital

- Blood transfusions, under certain circumstances

MEDICARE PART A COVERS ESSENTIALLY EVERYTHING ASSOCIATED WITH BEING IN THE HOSPITAL <u>EXCEPT PHYSICIANS' FEES</u>.

Private duty nurses are excluded. There are also some minor exclusions, such as a telephone or TV in your room (unless they're included in the hospital's fee, which they often are). The important noncovered expense is clearly doctors' fees, since multiple physicians, including surgeons, anesthesiologists, intensive care physicians, internists, and consulting specialists may be needed. This can become very costly, which is why having Medicare Part B, which pays doctors' fees, is so important for both outpatient *and* inpatient coverage.

⚠ **Medicare Part B is important for hospitalizations, not just office visits, because it covers physicians' fees <u>in and out of the hospital.</u>**

SKILLED NURSING FACILITY (SNF)

Medicare Part A covers up to 100 days in a skilled nursing facility, but *only* immediately after a "three-day minimum medically necessary hospital admission." This definition is critically important. The legislation empowering Medicare makes it very clear that Medicare is not meant to cover long-term nursing home care, also called *custodial care.*

⚠ **What most of us think of as "living in a nursing home" is simply not part of Medicare's responsibility.**

⚠ **Medicare will pay <u>nothing</u> toward an SNF admission that does not meet the following two requirements:**

- You were admitted to a hospital for at least 3 days.

- A physician has certified that the SNF is required for ongoing skilled treatment such as physical therapy, wound care, or intravenous medications.

When these criteria are met, Medicare Part A covers semiprivate rooms, meals, skilled nursing care, medications, and durable equipment used in the SNF, plus rehabilitative services such as physical, occupational, and speech therapy.

HOSPICE CARE

Hospice care is generally defined as palliative care—keeping the patient comfortable and controlling symptoms rather than attempting to "cure" a disease—for an individual with a terminal illness. For Medicare to cover the cost, the only specific requirement is that a physician certify that the patient is unlikely to live for more than six months. Many patients receiving hospice care have terminal cancer, but hospice can also be appropriate for other medical conditions. Medicare-approved hospice services are usually provided at home and may include physician and nursing visits, social work and counseling, home health aides, physical and occupational therapy, medications to control pain and other symptoms, and medical equipment such as a hospital bed. Coverage includes respite care, in which the patient can be admitted to an approved hospice facility for up to five days to allow the usual caregiver to rest.

HOME HEALTH SERVICES

For those who are homebound, Medicare Part A will cover certain specific home health services when provided by a Medicare-certified agency, including intermittent skilled nursing care, as well as physical, occupational, and speech therapy. The part-time assistance of a home health aide may be included, but full-time companions are not covered. A physician must certify that the individual is homebound and requires these services.

Chapter 10 contains extensive discussions of post-hospital skilled nursing facility stays, hospice care, and home health services.

Religious Nonmedical Health Care Institution (RNHCI)

Medicare defines this as "A facility that provides nonmedical healthcare items and services to people who need hospital or skilled nursing facility care, but for whom that care would be inconsistent with their religious beliefs." (http://www.medicare.gov/glossary/r.html) Medicare will cover the nonreligious portions of RNHCI care if the institution is certified by Medicare and the patient makes a written election that the choice of this type of care is based on religious beliefs. If you believe this relates to you, your religious organization can provide further information; or you can contact Medicare.

Who Qualifies for Medicare Part A and What Does It Cost?

Medicare Part A is the most basic part of Medicare and the easiest to understand. You qualify if you've reached your 65th birthday and you're a U.S. citizen or have been a legal U.S. resident for five years. For the majority of seniors, participating in Medicare Part A is free. Yes, FREE. Your income level, now or in the past, makes no difference.

THERE IS NO BETTER DEAL IN HEALTH CARE INSURANCE THAN
MEDICARE PART A.

Only one group of people must pay monthly premiums for Medicare Part A—those who have not paid FICA (Social Security) taxes for at least 10 years (40 quarters) and whose spouse has also not paid these taxes for at least 40 quarters. If either spouse has paid them, both qualify for premium-free Part A. The 40 quarters do *not* need to be consecutive. Paying FICA taxes for 30 quarters provides a partial discount off the full premium, but anything less than 30 quarters provides no cost reduction at all.

Widows and widowers can receive premium-free or reduced-premium Medicare Part A based on the FICA taxes paid by their deceased spouses. For those who've been divorced, it's more complicated. A divorced individual can qualify for premium-free or reduced-premium Medicare Part A based on a previous spouse's working record, but only if he or she was married to that person for a minimum of 10 years. Multiple marriages are not additive. Also, if a person is remarried at the time of applying for Medicare, an ex-spouse's FICA tax payments cannot be used to qualify for premium-free Part A.

⚠ **Don't expect to receive free or discounted Medicare Part A because your ex qualifies if you were not married to that one individual for at least 10 years or if you are currently remarried.**

In 2014, the full monthly premium for Medicare Part A is $441. For a person with 30 months of FICA taxes, it's $243 per month. These are substantial amounts and may be prohibitive for many seniors (a year of $441 monthly payments is $5,292).

And that's not all. As noted in Chapter 1, if you qualify to pay for Medicare Part A and don't sign up for it during your Initial Enrollment Period, penalties will result when you do enroll:

- Your Medicare Part A monthly premium goes up by 10%.

- It continues to be 10% higher for twice the number of years you delayed getting Part A.

For example, if you don't sign up for Medicare Part A for three years after you become eligible for it, your premium will have a 10% surcharge for six years.

If you qualify for free Part A, there's no penalty for not signing up during your Initial Enrollment Period, but you're turning down some very valuable benefits.

Even a short hospitalization can cost tens of thousands of dollars. What if you need to be admitted to a hospital multiple times? What if you're in the hospital for weeks? Anyone who qualifies for Medicare Part A and is contemplating not enrolling needs to consider very carefully the consequences of that decision. It may seem expensive if you don't qualify for premium-free coverage, but Medicare Part A provides incredible benefits. It's impossible for individuals age 65+ to buy less expensive hospital insurance, if they can find policies at all. Not getting Medicare Part A to avoid the monthly premium may prove to be an extremely costly mistake.

> FOR MOST OF US, SIGNING UP FOR MEDICARE PART A SHOULD BE A
> NO-BRAINER. HOSPITALIZATION REPRESENTS THE MOST EXPENSIVE PART OF
> MEDICAL CARE AND CAN RAPIDLY BANKRUPT THE UNINSURED.

Part A Cost Sharing

All parts of Medicare include some cost sharing. Your portion will be different for hospitals, skilled nursing facilities, hospice, and home care.

HOSPITAL

- For most hospital admissions, Medicare Part A cost sharing is simple: You are responsible for a deductible of $1,216 (for 2014), with *no additional cost sharing for the first 60 days in the hospital.*

- If you stay for more than 60 days, you become responsible for a copay of $304 per day for days 61–90 (maximum of $9,120).

- If you stay for more than 90 days, things get more complicated. Beyond 90 days, your copay increases to $608 per day. Additionally, hospitalization days beyond 90 are subject to what Medicare calls a **lifetime reserve** of 60 days. This means that Medicare Part A will cover only a *total* of 60 hospitalization days that extend beyond a 90-day stay, and the 60 days of coverage is a *maximum total for all hospitalizations over your lifetime.* Once you've used up the 60-day lifetime reserve you are responsible for the entire cost of any days beyond 90 in any hospitalization.

- There are situations in which you won't have to pay the $1,216 hospital deductible. With regard to inpatient care, Medicare defines a **benefit period** as starting on the first day of a hospital admission and ending when you have not received any hospital care or skilled nursing facility care for over 60 days. If you are readmitted (to the same hospital or a different one) within this benefit period, there is no second deductible. In fact, you can be in and out of the hospital multiple times, but as long as you're never home for more than 60 days, you remain in the same benefit period and have no new deductibles.

SKILLED NURSING FACILITY (SNF)

- For days 1–20 in an SNF, there is no cost sharing. Medicare covers 100% of the approved daily rate.

- For days 21–100, you have a copay of $152 per day (for 2014).

- There is no Medicare Part A coverage beyond 100 days.

- Benefit periods (as defined above) apply to SNFs and may, in fact, limit your coverage. The 100 days of Medicare-covered SNF care pertains to any given benefit period, not to a specific SNF admission. As a result, if you are admitted to a hospital twice during a given benefit period and each time you go to an SNF, there will be a *total* of 100 days of coverage for both SNF stays. Also, if the first SNF stay is longer than 20 days, you will begin paying the $152 daily copay on the first day of the second SNF stay.

HOSPICE

- Basic hospice care is free under Medicare Part A; no cost sharing.

- Prescription drugs required for pain management require a $5 copay.

- Physicians' fees are included if the doctor is paid by the hospice. Other doctors' fees are covered by Medicare Part B (minus your coinsurance).

- Respite care requires a coinsurance of 5% of the Medicare-approved cost.

- If a hospice patient requires hospitalization or emergency care for a nonhospice medical/surgical problem, normal Medicare Part A and Part B rules and cost sharing apply.

HOME HEALTH SERVICES

- No cost sharing for most home health services; Medicare pays 100%.

- Some items are covered by Medicare Part B, including certain durable medical equipment used in the home, with resultant 20% copays.

What If I Have Other Medical Insurance?

If you're paying for private medical insurance yourself, Medicare is virtually always a more cost-effective alternative. Think about it. With private insurance you are paying the entire premium. With Medicare, the U.S. government is paying a substantial part.

> MEDICARE PART A IS ALWAYS A BETTER DEAL THAN PRIVATE MEDICAL INSURANCE WHERE YOU (NOT AN EMPLOYER) ARE PAYING THE FULL PREMIUMS.

If you or your spouse is still working and you are receiving medical insurance from an employer, you will need to check on the specifics of how that insurance policy interacts with Medicare. Many policies will require you to have at least Medicare Part A once you reach age 65.

LARGE GROUP VS. SMALL GROUP POLICIES

▶ *If you're covered by a **large group** policy (20 or more insured individuals):* The private insurance is **primary,** paying first, with Medicare picking up some or all of the uncovered costs.

▶ *If you're covered by a **small group** policy (fewer than 20 insured individuals):* Medicare is primary, with claims going directly to Medicare and the private insurance company covering some or all of the cost sharing.

⚠ If you have small group employer-provided insurance, you MUST be enrolled in Medicare Part A and Medicare Part B.

Recommendation: If you have a large group policy and qualilfy for free Medicare Part A, sign up for at least Part A. Unless the private policy is unbelievably generous, the combination of private insurance plus Medicare Part A will provide more extensive inpatient coverage.

If you receive totally free medical benefits from an employer or union, it's clearly wise to keep those benefits. The combination of these private medical benefits plus Medicare will provide very comprehensive coverage. On the other hand, if your spouse is the employee and you have to pay for your portion of a family policy, it is often better to stop paying premiums and rely on Medicare. Your decision will depend on the specifics of the plan's coverage and its costs, which you'll have to compare to what Medicare provides and costs.

> CHECK WITH THE BENEFITS DEPARTMENT OF YOUR EMPLOYER OR UNION TO DETERMINE THE DETAILS OF YOUR EXISTING PLAN AND THEN DECIDE WHAT IS MOST COST-EFFECTIVE FOR YOU.

If you have retiree insurance and Medicare, Medicare *always* pays first, and the private insurance company pays second. The size of the group doesn't matter. As a result, you will definitely need Medicare—both Part A and Part B.

Health Savings Accounts and Medicare

There is one situation in which you cannot use Medicare Part A and private insurance at the same time—when your private insurance program involves the use of a Health Savings Account (HSA). In recent years, high-deductible insurance policies coupled with HSAs have become very popular with employers. Basically, the employer provides a medical insurance policy that does not begin paying benefits until a significant (perhaps $1,500) annual deductible has been met. In conjunction with the policy, the insured worker opens a Health Savings Account, into which the employer, the employee, or both can contribute pretax dollars. The funds in the HSA are then used to pay medical expenses. The exact details are not important here. If you have such a policy, you undoubtedly know it, since it functions very differently from typical medical insurance.

The important point is that *no contributions can be made to an HSA if you have Medicare*. Once you are receiving Medicare, you may continue to maintain a pre-existing HSA and use the money it contains to pay medical bills, but neither you nor your employer can contribute additional funds. Having Medicare Part A alone is sufficient to preclude such contributions. As a result, if your employer's health benefits program uses an HSA, you might be better off turning down that insurance and taking Medicare. Or you could find it advantageous to continue on your employer's plan and defer enrolling in Medicare Part A. You must check on the details of your plan and then compare the two options.

Key Points for Medicare Part A

- Medicare Part A covers inpatient care except doctors' fees.

- FREE for most seniors; premiums apply if neither the enrollee nor spouse has paid FICA taxes for 40 quarters.

- Widows/widowers can qualify based on former spouse's FICA payments; those who've been divorced may or may not, depending on years married and current marital status.

- Sign up during the Initial Enrollment Period or any subsequent General Enrollment Period. Late enrollment penalties apply only for those who must pay premiums—10% premium increase for twice the number of years enrollment is delayed.

- Having Medicare Part A along with an employer-sponsored plan may provide more complete inpatient coverage but is not allowed with an HSA plan.

- Hospital admission deductible is $1,216; no additional cost sharing for up to 60 days in the hospital.

- Hospitalizations beyond 60 days require daily copays; those beyond 90 days are subject to a lifetime reserve of 60 days.

- Subsequent hospital admissions may not have deductibles if within a single benefit period.

- Skilled nursing facility care covered only after a three-day hospital admission and limited to 100 days. Free for first 20 days, then daily copays of $152. Benefit periods apply.

- Minimal cost sharing for hospice care and home health care.

Bottom-Line Recommendations:

- Sign up for Medicare Part A as soon as you're eligible. It will almost always be the best deal you can get, no matter what your other insurance coverage.

- Get all the information you need from an employer's (yours or your spouse's) benefits administrator to determine whether you (or your spouse) should keep paying premiums for a private plan provided by the employer.

Chapter 3

Medicare Part B

"OK, now I see the catch. I do have to pay for Part B. How much? $104.90 a month. Not a bad price, but does it ever go on sale? How about coupons?"

What Does Medicare Part B Cover?

While Medicare Part A deals largely with inpatient costs, Medicare Part B covers primarily outpatient services. In addition, as already noted, doctors' fees are virtually always covered by Medicare Part B, whether inpatient or outpatient. For a listing of what Part B actually encompasses, see the following box.

WHAT MEDICARE PART B COVERS

- Doctors' fees, including primary care doctors and specialists, in and out of the hospital. Virtually any type of physician is covered for a Medicare-approved service. There is no limit on the number of different physicians you can see. With some exceptions, there are no limits on the number of visits with any particular physician.

- Wellness exams from your primary care doctor.

- Outpatient mental health care from psychiatrists, clinical psychologists, clinical social workers, and clinical nurse specialists.

- Free-standing outpatient (ambulatory) surgical centers.

- Emergency departments (ERs).

- Ambulances.

- Outpatient hospital services, such as diagnostic procedures or surgery done in a hospital setting.

- Clinical laboratory testing, including blood tests, urine tests, and cultures.

- X-ray studies and scans, including standard X-rays, CT scans, MRIs.

- Diagnostic tests such as electrocardiograms (EKGs).

- Kidney dialysis treatments.

- Chemotherapy given in a physician's office, clinic, or hospital outpatient department.

- Blood transfusions, with some limitations.

- Implantable pacemakers and defibrillators.

- Physical therapy, occupational therapy, speech therapy (with certain limitations).

- Counseling for tobacco cessation, obesity, & sexually transmitted diseases.

- Home health care (in combination with Part A coverage).

- Organ transplant services and associated immunosuppressive drugs.

- Durable medical equipment, such as wheelchairs, walkers, hospital beds, and oxygen equipment.

- Prosthetic devices, including artificial limbs and certain breast prostheses; neck, back, and limb braces.

- Diabetes testing supplies and diabetic self-management training.

- Certain specific screening tests:

  o Abdominal aneurysm screening

  o Bone density screening

  o Breast cancer screening—mammograms

- o Cardiovascular screening (blood fat levels)

- o Cervical cancer screening, including Pap tests

- o Colorectal cancer screening, including tests for blood in stool, sigmoidoscopy, colonoscopy

- o Diabetes screening

- o Depression screening

- o Glaucoma testing

- o HIV screening

- o Prostate cancer screening

- o Sexually transmitted infections

- Rehabilitative services:

- o Cardiac rehabilitation

- o Pulmonary rehabilitation

- Services of specific other doctors:

- o Foot exams and treatment by a podiatrist with some exceptions

- o Chiropractic care, but only to treat one specific spine condition

- o Optometry examinations and treatment for eye conditions and diseases

- Preventive services (immunizations):

- o Flu shots

- o Hepatitis B shots

- o Pneumococcal pneumonia shots

⚠️ **Outpatient services specifically NOT covered by Medicare Part B include dental care, dentures, hearing aids, routine eye care and glasses, acupuncture, and cosmetic surgery.**

Who Qualifies for Part B and What Does It Cost?

Just as with Medicare Part A, you qualify for Medicare Part B if you've reached age 65 and you either are a U.S. citizen or have been a legal resident of the United States for five years. How many years you paid Social Security tax (FICA) or Medicare tax doesn't matter.

Unlike Medicare Part A, however, Medicare Part B is not premium-free. Every recipient of Medicare Part B must pay at least the basic premium, which is $104.90 per month for 2014. Somewhat surprisingly, there was no increase from 2013 to 2014. In recent years, CMS had been raising the basic premium annually: It was $94.40 in 2011 and $99.90 in 2012. According to CMS, premiums cover approximately 25% of the cost of Medicare Part B, with the U.S. government using Medicare taxes and other revenues to pick up the other 75%. Presumably the basic premium will again begin to increase in the near future.

Higher-Income Medicare Recipients Pay More

More than 95% of all Medicare Part B participants pay only the basic monthly premium. However, Medicare enrollees with higher incomes are required to pay more for their Part B coverage (and also for their Part D drug coverage). Each individual's monthly premium is determined by what is known as **modified adjusted gross income** or **MAGI**, which is supplied to CMS by the Internal Revenue Service. This data is obtained from a person's most recently filed federal income tax return. For calculating 2014 premiums, for example, the most recent tax return was typically filed during 2013 and covers 2012.

Modified adjusted gross income is the sum of adjusted gross income plus tax-exempt income. To calculate MAGI, look at your federal tax return (Form 1040). Adjusted gross income is found on line 37 (at the bottom of the first page), and tax-exempt interest is found on line 8b (near the middle of the first page). Add them together and you've got MAGI. Note that this calculation does not include any of your tax deductions. It doesn't matter how much you deduct for mortgage interest, state taxes, charitable contributions, or anything else. Only *income* is used to determine your Medicare Part B and Part D premiums.

If MAGI is greater than $85,000 for an individual tax return or greater than $170,000 for a joint return, an additional Part B premium is charged. The following table, taken from Medicare's website, shows the 2014 monthly premiums for various MAGIs, both for taxpayers filing individually and for those filing jointly.

Part B Premiums by Income for 2014

If your modified adjusted gross income in 2012 was:		You Pay in 2014
File individual tax return	**File joint tax return**	
$85,000 or less	$170,000 or less	$104.90
above $85,000 up to $107,000	above $170,000 up to $214,000	$146.90
above $107,000 up to $160,000	above $214,000 up to $320,000	$209.80
above $160,000 up to $214,000	above $320,000 up to $428,000	$272.70
above $214,000	above $428,000	$335.70

Source: www.medicare.gov/your-medicare-costs/part-b-costs/part-b-costs.html

The table indicates that 2014 premiums are calculated from income data on the 2012 tax return, which is the most recently filed return. In fact, the amount you actually owe for premiums is determined by your current year's MAGI, not the MAGI two years ago. Since current year's income is unknown when you start paying your Medicare Part

B premiums in January, CMS uses the most recent data available from the IRS—and that's from two years ago. The assumption is that your income will remain constant, but that's not necessarily true, especially when you retire.

If you overpay, you will eventually receive a refund from CMS—a couple of years in the future. But if you are fairly certain that your income for the current year will be lower than it was two years ago, and that the difference will drop you into a lower premium category, you can request a lowered monthly premium based on your estimate of MAGI for the current year. This is done by calling Social Security (not Medicare) at 1-800-772-1213 and explaining the situation. You will be asked to complete and submit Form **SSA-44**, entitled "Medicare Income-Related Monthly Adjustment Amount – Life-Changing Event", which comes with detailed instructions.

Of course, when you ultimately file your tax return for the current year, CMS will check to see that your MAGI really was what you stated it would be. Should there be a discrepancy, CMS will require you to pay what you actually owe, possibly resulting in a substantial bill. If, during the current year, you realize that your income will be higher than expected and therefore your premiums have been too low, you can call Social Security and arrange to pay the additional amount.

How Do I Pay My Monthly Premium to CMS?

Easy. If you are receiving monthly Social Security benefit payments, your Part B premiums will be deducted from them. If you are not yet getting Social Security payments, you will be billed by CMS. You can pay these premiums in several ways, including direct debit from a bank account or by check. Your bill from CMS will explain your payment options.

Signing Up for Part B—and Failing to Do So

For those individuals who turn 65 and are already receiving Social Security or Railroad Retirement payments, Medicare will automatically sign you up for Medicare Part B, just as they will for Part A. You will receive a Medicare card that indicates you have both Part A and Part B coverage. If you're not yet receiving Social Security or Railroad Retirement benefits, you will have to sign up for Part B when you do so for Part A—during your Initial Enrollment Period.

What if you decide not to sign up for Medicare Part B during your Initial Enrollment Period? There are two possible scenarios.

▶ *If you simply don't want Medicare Part B and have no other insurance:* You will have to pay a very substantial penalty when you do eventually sign up. Specifically, for every full 12-month period you don't enroll after you're eligible, your Part B premium will increase by 10%, and these premium penalties will continue *indefinitely*. For example, if you delay enrolling for 48 months, your subsequent monthly premiums will be 140% of what they would otherwise be, for as long as you have Part B. If you live for 25 years after you finally enroll in Part B, you will have paid 40% more than you needed to for 25 years—simply because you delayed for four years.

⚠ **This is a huge penalty. Don't get ensnared by it. Feeling that you are healthy now and don't really need Medicare Part B coverage can cause your final expenditures for Part B to skyrocket. Choosing to save on Part B premiums for a few years is, in the long term, unwise.**

▶ *If you are covered by an insurance plan based on "current employment"* (either you or your spouse may be the employee): You qualify for the Special Enrollment Period discussed in Chapter 1, which runs for eight months after the month that employment terminates or the employer's health plan ends. Signing up for Medicare Part B during this period will result in no penalties being assessed.

There is also, however, the plan size to consider:

▶ *If your employer-sponsored plan has fewer than 20 enrollees:* Medicare is the primary payer, with the private insurance plan only supplementing Medicare. For this reason, the plan sponsor can require you to enroll in both Part A and Part B so you'll have the needed Medicare coverage.

▶ *If your employer-sponsored plan has 20 or more enrollees:* It will be the primary payer, and because you might then be covered sufficiently, your signing up for Part B is optional. You are allowed to defer enrolling in Medicare Part B and thereby avoid the monthly premium, but be aware that the result might be incomplete coverage for physicians and outpatient care. Assuming that the large plan is creditable (and you'll need to get documentation of this from the insurance company), you will be entitled to a Special Enrollment Period when your participation ends.

⚠️ You do NOT qualify for a Special Enrollment Period if your private insurance plan is a retiree insurance plan or COBRA. Be careful not to be trapped into paying indefinite penalties because you didn't realize your retiree health plan or COBRA would not qualify you for a Special Enrollment Period.

SHOULD YOU EVER KEEP YOUR RETIREE OR COBRA PLAN ONCE YOU'RE ELIGIBLE FOR MEDICARE?

▶ *If you have a particularly generous retiree plan* (uncommon in recent years): You might consider keeping it when you enroll in Medicare Part B because you'll have more comprehensive coverage than Part B alone.

▶ *If you are paying for COBRA,* which is extremely expensive: There is almost no circumstance where it is advisable to delay Medicare Part B or even to continue paying for COBRA while on Medicare.

Chapter 4 will show you how to augment Medicare Parts A and B coverage for a much lower cost than COBRA by purchasing a Medigap plan.

A note regarding TRICARE (medical insurance for active-duty military, retirees, and families): If you are a military retiree, you must enroll in Medicare Part B and pay premiums (along with free Part A) to keep your TRICARE coverage. Rules are different for active-duty military and their dependents, so check with TRICARE regarding your specific situation.

Part B Cost Sharing

Cost sharing under Part B has two components:

1. An annual deductible, which is modest:

   For 2014, you must pay $147 for Part B services before Medicare pays anything; after that, Medicare begins to pay its portion of every covered service.

2. <u>Coinsurance and copays, which are much more significant:</u>

> For the vast majority of Medicare Part B services, you are responsible for 20% of Medicare's approved fee. What does this mean? For every service covered by Part B, CMS establishes a specific approved fee. Many factors go into determining this amount, including the complexity of the service, who provides it, in what setting it occurs (office, home, operating room, etc.), and materials required. There are also geographic variations related to the costs of doing business in various parts of the country. The calculations used are complex. In the end, every covered service receives a Medicare-approved fee for every geographic locality. For most services covered by Part B, Medicare then pays 80% of the approved fee. The other 20% is your responsibility—your coinsurance.

> Some services covered by Part B have specific copays, especially those obtained in hospital outpatient departments. These will vary, and you will have to inquire about the specific copays applicable to the tests and procedures you receive.

CRITICAL CONCEPTS: ACCEPTING ASSIGNMENT AND PARTICIPATING PROVIDERS

To determine your costs for Medicare Part B services, you need to fully understand the concept of **accepting assignment**. The Medicare-approved fee for any service may not be the provider's regular fee. In most cases, it's not. In general, Medicare-approved fees are *lower than* providers' regular fees, often substantially so. If a provider (physician, laboratory, etc.) agrees to accept the Medicare-approved fee as full payment for a service, then the provider has "accepted assignment." Medicare will pay its portion, and you will pay your cost sharing portion, but the total amount the provider receives will only be the Medicare-approved fee.

Providers who agree to accept assignment *all the time* are known as **participating providers**. Others may choose to accept assignment only under certain circumstances, such as for specific patients or specific procedures. Participating providers, on the other hand, acknowledge that Medicare's approved fee is the maximum amount they will receive for *every* service they provide to *every* Medicare patient. They will always bill Medicare directly for the 80% that Medicare pays and will charge you the 20% coinsurance.

> **Participating provider:** A provider that agrees to charge only the Medicare-approved fee for all services.
>
> **Non-participating provider:** A provider that sees Medicare patients and sends bills to Medicare but <u>does not</u> accept Medicare's approved fee as full payment for the service and may charge up to Medicare's limiting charges.

NON-PARTICIPATING PROVIDERS—WHAT'S UP WITH THEM?

What if your physician is non-participating? Does that mean that he won't see Medicare patients and won't bill Medicare for his services? Absolutely not. The concept of the non-participating provider is one of the most widely misunderstood features of Medicare. A non-participating provider *does* see Medicare patients and *does* submit claims to Medicare on behalf of his patients. He does not, however, accept Medicare-approved fees as his full fees. And he does not accept assignment on a regular basis.

The term *non-participating* is a terrible one, since it implies that a non-participating provider wants nothing to do with Medicare. But that's not the case. There are, in fact, some physicians who totally reject dealing with Medicare. I'll talk about them later, but they are *not* what Medicare calls non-participating physicians. It's important to be very clear on this point.

So if a non-participating physician does not accept Medicare's fees as her full fees, can she charge you as much as she wants? No. There are very definite restrictions on how much she can charge. Medicare accomplishes this by creating what's called a **limiting charge**. Here's how it works. For all services by non-participating providers, Medicare lowers its Medicare-approved fee by 5%. Thus, the approved fee for a non-participating doctor is only 95% of the fee for a doctor who participates. Medicare then allows the non-participating provider to charge you 115% of the lowered (95%) charge. Multiplying 95% times 115% comes out to 109.25%.

As a result, the limiting charge, which is the maximum amount you can be charged, is only 9.25% higher than Medicare's approved fee. In cases like this, the provider charges you the entire limiting fee and must submit a claim to Medicare on your behalf. Medicare then reimburses you based on the reduced (95%) approved fee. More specifically, Medicare pays its usual 80% but pays it only on the reduced (95%) fee. 95% times 80% equals 76%, so you receive 76% of the Medicare-approved fee. Your out-of-pocket cost is the difference between the limiting fee (which you owe the physician) and the amount that Medicare reimburses you.

If you think this is incredibly complicated, you're absolutely right. It causes widespread confusion among patients and providers alike. You would be shocked to know how many physicians don't truly understand how the Medicare Part B payment system actually works.

To try to clarify things, let's look at a specific example:

> *Jim Wong goes to see a medical specialist for a heart problem. The doctor's normal fee for the visit is $150, but Medicare's approved fee is $100. Let's assume Jim has already met his $147 annual Medicare Part B deductible for the year.*

IF THE DOCTOR IS A PARTICIPATING PROVIDER:		IF THE DOCTOR IS NON-PARTICIPATING:		
Regular fee	$150.00	Regular fee		$150.00
Approved fee	$100.00	Approved fee	(95% of $100)	$ 95.00
Medicare pays 80%	$80.00	Limiting fee	(115% of $95)	$109.25
Jim pays (20 % coinsurance)	$20.00	Jim pays the doctor		$109.25
		Medicare reimburses Jim (95% of $80)		$76.00
		Jim's cost ($109.25 – $76.00)		$33.25

You can observe several important points from this example:

- The physician's regular fee doesn't matter; Medicare's approved fee always serves as the basis for calculating the final fee.

- Medicare pays out less for non-participating providers (only 95% as much).

- The maximum amount a non-participating provider can receive is only 109.25% of the Medicare-approved fee.

- A patient's out-of-pocket costs are 66.25% more for a non-participating physician. In this example, Jim pays $33.25 for non-participating services and $20.00 for participating services. ($33.25 minus $20 = $13.25; divided by $20 = 66.25%). This percentage will pertain to all Medicare-approved services. Here it was only $13.25. In other cases, in which bills get large, the difference between what is paid to a participating provider and a non-participating one can be significant. If Medicare's approved fee for the service had been $1,000 rather than $100, the difference in out-of-pocket cost would have been $132.50.

On occasion, a non-participating provider may choose to accept assignment. Perhaps he's known a patient for a long time or feels a particular patient needs a financial break. If he does this, he actually makes less money than a participating provider. Here's why. Since he's non-participating, his Medicare fee is only 95% of the regular Medicare-approved fee. In Jim's case, described above, that would be $95. Medicare pays 80% of the $95 ($76) and Jim pays 20% of the $95 ($19). The physician receives a total of $95, which is $5 less than a participating provider would get. This is why non-participating physicians accept assignment only infrequently. A physician who accepts assignment fairly often is better off becoming a participating provider.

Bottom-line cost to you in using a participating vs. non-participating provider: Your out-of-pocket expense can be up to <u>66.25% higher when using a non-participating provider.</u>

Still, you may feel it's worth the extra cost to seek services from a non-participating doctor or facility that you prefer.

In Chapter 4 you'll learn about a way to make your cost for seeing a non-participating provider equal the cost for a participating one.

SOMETIMES MEDICARE PART B PAYS 100%

Some services covered by Medicare Part B do not require cost sharing. In such cases, Medicare pays the entire fee if the services are received from a participating provider. Most involve preventive care. Only recently has Medicare altered its rules to encompass and even emphasize wellness and prevention. Now, during the first 12 months that you are enrolled in Medicare Part B, you are entitled to a free "Welcome to Medicare" preventive care visit with your doctor. The focus of this visit is creating a plan, based on your particular risk factors and lifestyle, to keep you healthy. Subsequently, you may have one free "Wellness" visit each year to modify the plans developed earlier. Keep in mind, however, that these "Wellness" exams are very definitely *not* comprehensive physical exams. Appendix A contains a discussion of what's really included in a "Welcome to Medicare" exam. Other services, such as laboratory tests or additional examinations, may be provided at the time of a "Wellness" visit, and cost sharing may apply.

Other preventive services also require no cost sharing: certain screening tests for breast cancer, cervical cancer, colorectal cancer, prostate cancer, HIV, diabetes, and blood lipid (fat) levels, as well as immunizations for hepatitis B, pneumococcal pneumonia, and influenza (flu). Your physician must be participating for these screening tests and immunizations to be free.

⚠ **Determining whether each physician, facility, laboratory, or supplier accepts assignment is *your* responsibility. Ideally you should be told when you make your appointment, but mistakes happen. Ask!**

Doctors Who Are Beyond Non-participating

You may encounter some providers who want nothing to do with Medicare at all. They will generally be physicians who feel that Medicare's limiting fees are too low and won't accept them. Unfortunately, Medicare has no name for these physicians, which is why confusion arises so readily with the term *non-participating physician*. We can call them "physicians who reject Medicare" if you like. You are free to see a provider of this type, but you must be aware that Medicare will pay *nothing* toward the cost of these services. Don't believe anyone who tells you that you might be able to get some reimbursement from Medicare. *The facts are simple: If a provider charges you more than the Medicare limiting fee, you will get nothing back from Medicare.* You will have to sign what's called a **private contract** with this type of provider, agreeing to pay the full amount yourself. The provider must inform you whether or not the services would be covered by Medicare if you received them from a provider who sees Medicare patients. You can never be asked to sign a private contract for emergency care.

Does It Matter Where I See a Doctor or Have a Procedure Done?

You bet it does. And the cost differences can be tremendous.

Outpatient services covered by Medicare Part B can be obtained in a variety of settings, including a physician's office, an ambulatory surgical center, or a hospital outpatient department. If you see a doctor in his office, whether for a medical visit, diagnostic procedure, or minor surgery, you will be responsible only for the cost sharing applicable to the doctor's fee.

By contrast, if you receive medical, surgical, or certain diagnostic services in a hospital outpatient department or ambulatory surgical center, there will be a second charge with additional cost sharing. A trip to the hospital emergency room will result in two separate fees or sets of fees. You (and Medicare) will be charged by the physicians who treat you and by the emergency facility. Many surgical procedures require a free-standing ambulatory surgical center or a hospital outpatient surgical suite; anesthesia may be needed. In these cases, you will again be charged separately by the surgeon, the anesthesiologist, and the facility. The same holds true for diagnostic studies that sometimes utilize special procedure rooms or equipment, such as colonoscopies.

Since all of these situations are purely outpatient, all components are covered solely by Medicare Part B. However, cost sharing for facility charges is often handled very differently from cost sharing for doctors. For a free-standing ambulatory surgical center, you are generally responsible for 20% coinsurance, just like a doctor. But when utilizing a hospital outpatient department, whether the service is an emergency room visit, ambulatory surgery, or a diagnostic procedure, you will have a specific *copay* for the hospital facility, the size of which will vary greatly according to what was done.

A copay of this type cannot exceed $1,216. Does this number look familiar? You've seen it before. It is exactly the same amount as the Medicare Part A deductible for a hospitalization of up to 60 days. *In other words, your cost sharing obligation for a single outpatient procedure could be as great as the cost sharing for a prolonged and complicated hospital stay.* Outpatient copays of this type apply to *each procedure separately.* Every time you're back in the hospital's outpatient diagnostic facility getting a biopsy or an endoscopy or a scan, there will be a separate Part B copay. As a result, multiple diagnostic and/or surgical procedures can result in very substantial costs to you.

The implications of these hospital outpatient copays are great. In the first place, for any elective procedure or test you should find out ahead of time what the copay will be. In an emergency situation this will not be possible, but if you have the time, knowing your costs may well save you from an extremely unpleasant surprise. Secondly, many medical and minor surgical visits can often be done in a doctor's office as well as in a more complex facility. Sewing up a simple laceration is an example. Performing a skin biopsy and removing a cinder from your eye are others. Many times going to a doctor's office about a headache, belly pain, or cough is much more cost effective than going to the emergency room. In this sense, an Immediate Care Center is considered a doctor's office. You clearly must make decisions based on factors other than cost alone, but you should definitely be aware of the price you pay for utilizing complex medical facilities.

Does Original Medicare Place Any Limitations on Services?

In general, Original Medicare (versus Medicare Advantage) allows you to see any physician of your choice and, in most cases, as often as needed. Always keep in mind, though, that all services covered by Medicare must be "medically necessary" and an audit by CMS or a local CMS contractor could determine that the services were excessive.

For certain services, however, Medicare has begun to impose specific limits. A notable example involves physical therapy, occupational therapy, and speech therapy. For 2014, Medicare allows $1,920 for physical therapy and speech therapy combined. Since Medicare pays approximately $100 per hour for therapy, this comes to roughly 19 hours. Once the $1,920 limit has been reached, the therapist can request additional sessions up to a total of $3,700 ($1,920 + $1,780 more). Thereafter, the case must be specifically reviewed. Similar limits apply to occupational therapy. No specific number of visits is guaranteed for payment. In all cases the patient must exhibit "functional improvement in a reasonable and predictable amount of time" or the therapy must be terminated.

Medicare also has restrictions on where you can purchase or rent durable medical equipment. In much of the United States, you can use any Medicare-approved supplier, all of which must agree to accept assignment. Now Medicare has established a Competitive Bidding Program in nine test areas around the country. When expanded, this program will require getting durable medical equipment from specific suppliers that have submitted successful bids to Medicare. A similar program has been instituted for diabetes testing supplies obtained by mail. As of July 1, 2013, all such supplies have to be obtained from a Medicare contract supplier.

Restrictions of the types described above will assuredly become more common in coming years as pressures increase to control Medicare costs. You'll hear about them as they happen. Stay tuned.

Key Points for Medicare Part B

- **Medicare Part B covers outpatient care and all doctors' fees.**

- **Premiums required of everyone; higher premiums for those whose modified adjusted gross income (MAGI) exceeds $85,000 for single taxpayers or $170,000 for joint filers.**

- **Enroll during the Initial Enrollment Period or any Special Enrollment Period if previously covered by creditable insurance based on current employment (not a retirement plan).**

- **Failing to enroll at the proper time involves a penalty of 10% for every 12-month period you delay enrolling; penalties continue every year indefinitely.**

- **Physicians who accept assignment agree to accept Medicare's fee schedule for all Medicare patients; Medicare pays 80% and the patient 20%.**

- **Physicians who don't accept assignment can charge up to Medicare's limiting fee—109.25% of the Medicare approved fee. Medicare reimburses 80% of 95% of the Medicare fee, which is 76%, while patient pays the difference between 109.25% and 76%.**

- Participating providers agree to accept assignment all the time; non-participating providers may accept assignment some of the time.

- Physicians who refuse to see any patients under Medicare must have each patient sign a private contract. No Medicare reimbursement at all.

- Medicare pays 100% for designated preventive services.

- 20% coinsurance applies to many outpatient services such as laboratory tests, diagnostic procedures, and surgery, but hospital outpatient services may have copays as high as $1,216. Each test or procedure will have a separate copay or coinsurance.

- Medicare is beginning to restrict the number of visits for certain services, so far mainly physical/occupational/speech therapy.

- Restrictions on where one can obtain durable medical equipment and diabetes testing supplies have begun.

Bottom-Line Recommendations:

- Be sure to sign up for Medicare Part B during the applicable enrollment period to avoid lifelong penalties in premiums.

- Don't put off enrolling in Part B because you currently have retiree or COBRA insurance; you might, however, benefit from keeping retiree insurance while you're enrolled in Part B if your private coverage is excellent—it may provide greater total benefits.

- Be prepared to pay close attention to where you obtain services since your choice of doctors (participating, non-participating, or rejecting Medicare altogether) and facilities (doctor's office/clinic vs. hospital) can make a major difference in your out-of-pocket costs.

Chapter 4

Medicare Supplement Insurance Policies (Medigap Plans)

"Hold everything. Having Medicare-approved fees is pretty nifty, but what can we do about that nasty 20% coinsurance every time I see a doctor? The cost sharing is killing me."

Insurance to Cover Cost Sharing

You've just read all about Medicare Parts A and B, including what they cover and your costs. It should be clear by now that coverage is very comprehensive, but that deductibles, copays, and coinsurance can result in substantial out-of-pocket costs to you. In particular, the 20% coinsurance for doctor bills and the copays for outpatient hospital services can add up quickly. Are there any ways to mitigate these expenses? The answer is yes:

- **Small-group employer-sponsored insurance** will be secondary to Medicare and may cover much of your cost sharing obligations.

- **Retiree insurance** may pay for some or all of what Medicare doesn't.

- Those on **Medicaid** plus Medicare will find that the combined programs provide virtually full coverage.

But if none of these applies to you, you can purchase what's known as a **Medicare Supplement Insurance Policy,** more commonly known as a **Medigap Policy.** We'll call it Medigap from here on for brevity.

A Medigap policy is an insurance plan sold and administered by a private insurance company under strict Medicare guidelines. *These policies are specifically designed to fill in cost sharing gaps in Original Medicare Parts A and B. They do not work with any other types of medical insurance.* Specifically, they do <u>not</u> cover any of the cost sharing in Medicare Part D (drug benefit) or in Medicare Part C (Medicare Advantage plans).

What Do Medigap Policies Cover?

Insurance companies selling Medigap policies must follow specific federal parameters and also comply with state laws. They can issue only what are called "standardized" Medigap policies, each of which provides a very specific set of coverages. The following table, taken directly from Medicare literature and websites (with slight modifications for clarity), describes what these policies cover. To choose the policy that's best for you, you'll need to understand how the 10 lettered plans compare.

Along the top of the table, the different available **Medigap Plans** are indicated by CAPITAL LETTERS. Medicare has used the letters A through N to name each of the standardized policies, but plans E, H, I, and J can no longer be purchased. Along the left side of the table, under the heading **Medigap Benefits,** are nine different distinct benefits that Medigap policies can provide. *YES* means a benefit is fully covered; a % means it's covered up to that percentage; an empty box indicates the benefit is not covered.

The best way to start untangling this complicated table is to get a solid grasp of what's covered by each of the nine benefits (see pages 50-52). Then the rest of the table becomes much easier to figure out.

Medicare Supplement Insurance (Medigap) Plans

Medigap Benefits	Medigap				Plans					
	A	B	C	D	F*	G	K	L	M	N
1. Part A daily copays; hospital per diem costs for up to 365 additional days beyond the lifetime reserve	YES	YES	YES	YES	YES	YES	YES	YES	YES	YES
2. Part B coinsurance and copays	YES	YES	YES	YES	YES	YES	50%	75%	YES	YES***

Medigap Benefits	Medigap	Plans								
	A	B	C	D	F*	G	K	L	M	N
3. Blood (first three pints)	YES	YES	YES	YES	YES	YES	50%	75%	YES	YES
4. Part A hospice care coinsurance and copays	YES	YES	YES	YES	YES	YES	50%	75%	YES	YES
5. Skilled nursing facility copays			YES	YES	YES	YES	50%	75%	YES	YES
6. Part A deductibles		YES	YES	YES	YES	YES	50%	75%		YES
7. Part B annual deductible			YES		YES					
8. Part B excess charges					YES	YES				
9. Foreign travel emergency (up to plan limits)			YES	YES	YES	YES			YES	YES
Out-of-pocket limit**	N/A	N/A	N/A	N/A	N/A	N/A	$4,800	$2,400	N/A	N/A

*Plan F is also offered in a high-deductible form. If you choose this option, you must pay for Medicare cost sharing up to the $2,140 deductible (for 2014) before the Medigap plan pays anything.

**After you meet your out-of-pocket yearly limit and your yearly Part B deductible, the Medigap plans pays 100% of cost sharing for the rest of the calendar year.

***Plan N pays 100% of the Part B coinsurance, except for a copay of up to $20 for some office visits and up to a $50 copay for emergency room visits that don't result in an admission.

Medigap Policy Benefits

1. *Medicare Part A Daily Copays and Hospital Per Diem Costs (up to an additional 365 days after Medicare benefits have been used up)*

    As discussed in Chapter 2, the first 60 days of a hospital admission are 100% covered by Medicare after the $1,216 Part A deductible; there are *no* daily copays during this period. For a hospital stay longer than 60 days, you must pay a $304 daily copay for days 61–90; for days 91 and beyond, you must pay a $608 daily copay—but remember that there is a 60-day lifetime reserve on hospital stays longer than 90 days. Once you've used up that reserve, you are responsible for the *entire* daily hospital rate every day you're there. This Medigap benefit picks up the $304 per day and the $608 per day. Even more important, it pays 100% of hospital daily charges for another 365 days beyond the 60-day lifetime reserve.

2. *Medicare Part B Coinsurance and Copays*

    This benefit pays all coinsurance and copays for Medicare-approved Part B services, including the 20% coinsurance typical of most physician fees, laboratory tests, procedures, therapy of various kinds, and durable medical equipment. It also covers the copays, which can be up to $1,216 per service, for outpatient surgery or diagnostic procedures performed in a hospital outpatient department.

3. *Blood (First 3 Pints)*

    This benefit pays for the three pints of blood that Medicare Part A and Part B do not cover.

4. *Part A Hospice Care Coinsurance or Copays*

    Cost sharing is minimal for hospice care, but this benefit covers those costs.

5. *Skilled Nursing Facility Copays*

    Medicare Part A covers 100% of the first 20 days in a skilled nursing facility. This benefit covers the $152 per day that you must pay for days 21–100. There is no coverage whatsoever beyond 100 days. An SNF admission must occur directly after a hospital admission of three or more days.

⚠ This benefit provides <u>no coverage for long-term, custodial nursing home stays.</u>

6. *Medicare Part A Deductible*

This benefit pays the $1,216 deductible for each hospitalization or "benefit period" as defined in the discussion of Medicare Part A.

> A PLAN THAT INCLUDES BENEFITS #1 AND #6 WILL PROVIDE TOTAL COVERAGE FOR ALMOST ANY HOSPITAL ADMISSION.

7. *Medicare Part B Deductible*

The $147 annual deductible is covered by this benefit.

8. *Medicare Part B Excess Charges*

This benefit pertains specifically to charges from providers who do not accept assignment (non-participating providers). It covers the excess amount charged by the provider up to the limiting fee (109.25% of the Medicare-approved fee), which is the maximum amount the provider can expect to receive.

> THIS MAY BE AN IMPORTANT BENEFIT FOR YOU IF YOU PLAN TO STICK WITH PROVIDERS WHO YOU KNOW ARE NON-PARTICIPATING, OR YOU SIMPLY WANT THE FLEXIBILITY TO SEE ANY DOCTOR WHO SEES MEDICARE PATIENTS.

9. *Foreign Travel Emergency*

Original Medicare pays for emergency medical services in foreign countries only under very rare circumstances. You should assume you have no Medicare coverage outside the

United States. The Foreign Travel Emergency benefit will reimburse you for 80% of the costs of hospitals, physicians, and related care in foreign countries, but only for emergency services of the kind that would normally be covered in the United States The emergency must begin within the first 60 days of your trip. There is a $250 calendar year deductible and a $50,000 lifetime limit.

THIS CAN BE A USEFUL BENEFIT IF YOU DO A LOT OF TRAVELING.

Comparing Plans

Obviously you have lots of choices, and you'll need to decide which of the nine Medigap benefits are important to you and what you can afford. To start, notice that all lettered Medigap Plans include the first four benefits. Plan F, which includes all nine benefits, is also available in a high-deductible form.

Be aware, however, that you may not have quite as many choices as it appears. State laws and the insurance companies that underwrite plans in a given geographic area will determine which lettered plans are available. By federal law, any company selling Medigap policies must offer Plan A and may offer others. If a company sells any plan in addition to Plan A, its offerings must include either Plan C or Plan F. Beyond those rules, each company can determine which plans it chooses to sell in any locale.

In analyzing the plans, consider the following:

- Even the most basic one, Plan A, provides a lot of coverage. The 365 days of additional hospital coverage (benefit #1) can be invaluable if you have many long hospitalizations.

- Picking up Part B procedure copays and 20% doctor coinsurance (benefit #2) can save you a huge amount of money if you become ill and have to see multiple doctors and get many tests. As you will learn later, some short hospitalizations are not considered admissions by Medicare and are classified as outpatient care. The coinsurance and copays associated with this type of hospitalization are paid by benefit #2.

- The first two Medigap Policy benefits provide the core of Medigap coverage. Beyond these two, you are adding benefits that you may or may not feel are worth an additional premium. For example, if you have a chronic illness for which SNF stays are likely to be needed after hospitalizations, select a plan that includes benefit #5.

- The 50% and 75% coverage characteristic of Plans K and L make them somewhat cumbersome to use. They provide some cost savings, but their premiums may not differ much from Plan A.

The Cadillac of Medigap

The most comprehensive Medigap Plans are F and G. They differ from each other only in coverage of the $147 annual Medicare Part B deductible. What separates these two plans from all the others, however, is that they are the only plans that cover your coinsurance when you see non-participating providers. As noted above, this means they are most valuable to you if you specifically want coverage for physicians and other providers who don't accept Medicare assignment. If you have a Medigap Plan F or G, the insurance company will subsequently reimburse you for the remainder of what you paid the non-participating provider; you will ultimately have no out-of-pocket expense. Many of our fellow Medicare recipients must believe that Excess Charges coverage is important, since Plan F is the most widely owned type of Medigap policy nationwide.

WITH A MEDIGAP PLAN F, YOU WILL HAVE NO OUT-OF-POCKET COSTS FOR ANY PARTICIPATING OR NON-PARTICIPATING PROVIDERS THAT YOU USE.

You may—or may not—have to submit a claim to the Medigap insurance carrier after you receive your payment from Medicare, which can require some paperwork on your part. When you have a Plan F or G, some non-participating providers will bill Medicare and then bill your Medigap insurance carrier for you, since they know they will receive the entire limiting fee by doing so; some won't.

⚠ Plans F and G do NOT pay anything toward the costs of using a provider who rejects Medicare altogether. Do not let anyone tell you that a Medigap Plan F or Plan G will help to pay for services rendered under a private contract. It's simply not true.

The Case for Cadillac Lite (High-Deductible Plan F)

Take particular note of the high-deductible Plan F. This choice has all the coverage of regular Plan F, but there is a $2,140 annual deductible (for 2014). This means that you must pay the first $2,140 of the cost sharing charges that the regular Plan F normally covers. Because of the comprehensive benefits, the $2,140 will be your maximum out-of-pocket cost. But why expose yourself to that extra expense? Because this plan generally costs substantially less than all the other Medigap plans. I have seen it available for a monthly premium as low as $35—a small fraction of a regular Plan F policy. This plan may be a good choice for you if you cannot afford a higher premium and will settle for a safety net. But it might even be a superior option if you *can* afford the regular Plan F. Here's why:

> Assume you can find a high-deductible Plan F for $35 per month, which comes to $420 per year. Were you to use up your entire $2,140 deductible, your total cost for the year would be $420 + $2,140 = $2,560. If a regular Plan F cost $210 monthly, the annual premium would be $2,520. Thus, at the end of the year, the total costs for both options are similar. However, if in any given year you don't have many medical expenses and don't use up your $2,140 deductible, then the high-deductible Plan F becomes the much less expensive option.

The example above uses rates presently available in southeastern Connecticut. Just across the state line in metropolitan New York City rates are higher, but the high-deductible Plan F fares even better. There the least expensive high-deductible Plan F, at the time of this writing, costs $64 per month and the least expensive Plan F about $257. So the annual costs are $768 and $3,000 respectively. Adding the $2,140 deductible to the $768 annual premium comes to $2,908, which is actually less than the cost of a regular Plan F.

Obviously, the validity of this comparison depends on how much you pay for the regular Plan F versus the high-deductible version. Relative costs will vary considerably by locality. It's definitely worth considering.

⚠ If you believe you'll have difficulty dealing with the complexities of medical billing, you might want to avoid the high deductible version. Any plan that has deductibles or provides partial coverage will result in a lot more paperwork for you. With a regular Plan F, 100% of your Medicare-related expenses should be covered. Any attempts by hospitals or other providers to charge you additional amounts will be obvious and easy for you to question/challenge. It's much more difficult to reconcile what you're being charged when you have to evaluate a series of bills for coinsurance and copays. In particular, bills from hospitals can be lengthy and confusing, with page after page of codes and little written explanation. It's very easy to be overwhelmed and overcharged.

State Laws and Medigap

As noted above, state laws will often determine which lettered Medigap plans are available and will impose restrictions that affect prices. For example, in some states Medigap carriers must sell the same Plan A policies to seniors and to Medicare recipients on disability, which can result in Plan A policies being disproportionately expensive. Three states—Massachusetts, Minnesota, and Wisconsin—have available Medigap options different from those of other states. Residents of these three states should contact their State Insurance Assistance Program (SHIP) for a listing of available plans along with the insurance companies that are selling them.

In some states, a less expensive Medigap variant known as Medicare SELECT is available. Medicare SELECT plans are similar to regular Medigap plans, but they require you to use only certain hospitals and/ or doctors to be covered (except in emergencies). As you know, Original Medicare imposes no restrictions on which providers you may use. Medicare SELECT plans add restrictions, but only to the cost sharing portion. Such plans add an element of managed care and generally cost less than comparable Medigap plans.

When Should I Apply for a Medigap Policy?

All Medigap policies are sold by private insurance companies. Medicare regulations allow these companies to utilize **medical underwriting** in deciding whether to insure you, in determining how much to charge you, and in excluding any pre-existing conditions for a period of time. Medical underwriting means that the company looks at your medical history, including illnesses, operations, ongoing medical conditions, lifestyle, and family history, to determine how great a financial risk insuring you might be. As a result, you can be charged more or denied coverage entirely based on your health. However, if you apply for a Medigap policy during what's called your **Medigap Open Enrollment Period**, you can minimize or even entirely avoid the effects of medical underwriting. That's why it's extremely important to buy a Medigap policy at the correct time.

As many of you undoubtedly know, the Affordable Care Act (ObamaCare) prevents pre-existing conditions from being used to deny coverage or influence premiums. This does not, however, appear to apply to Medigap policies.

THE MEDIGAP OPEN ENROLLMENT PERIOD

⚠️ It's important to buy Medigap insurance during the Medigap Open Enrollment Period. If you do, you <u>cannot be rejected,</u> you <u>cannot be charged more than the company's base rate</u> for that plan, and <u>any pre-existing conditions must be covered</u> (although coverage may be delayed on those conditions for up to six months).

Your Medigap Open Enrollment Period is defined as the six-month period that starts on the first day of the month you're at least 65 years old *and enrolled in Medicare Part B*. As you know, you don't have to enroll in Part B at the same time as Part A if you have other, creditable insurance coverage. It's when you sign up for Medicare Part B that counts.

▶ *If you apply for a Medigap policy during this Medigap Open Enrollment Period:* The insurance company *must* accept you and can charge you only its base rate, no matter what health conditions you may have. You must be charged exactly the same amount as someone with no medical problems at all. Pre-existing conditions cannot be excluded from coverage under the policy. The insurance company does have the right to delay covering any pre-existing condition for a period of six months, but only if that condition was diagnosed or treated during the previous six months. Older medical conditions cannot be excluded or limited. Once the Medigap policy has been in force for six months, *all* pre-existing conditions become fully covered. The advantages of applying during the Medigap Open Enrollment Period are clearly substantial. This cannot be overstated.

▶ *If you apply for a Medigap policy during the Open Enrollment Period and you had other medical insurance prior to applying:* It's even better. In this case, there may be a shorter pre-existing conditions waiting period (i.e., less than six months) or none at all. Your previous insurance must be creditable coverage. The insurance carrier for the prior plan can tell you whether it is creditable and provide you with documentation. If you had creditable insurance coverage for six months, and had no gap in coverage of more than 63 days, then *all waiting periods are eliminated.* You will be fully covered with no exceptions from day one.

Here are some examples that may make these rules clearer.

- Dwayne Robinson just turned 65 and is enrolling in Medicare Parts A and B. He lost his regular job and his insurance two years ago; currently he works part-time. He has high blood pressure for which he takes two medicines. Dwayne is thrilled that he can now get medical coverage under Medicare. He wants a Medigap plan, finds one that he can afford, and applies for it two weeks after starting Medicare. He gets the policy, although treatment of his blood pressure (but nothing else) is excluded for six months.

- Millie Yarborough has been covered by her husband's employer-sponsored medical insurance plan, but she has to pay a lot for it. She feels Medicare will provide better value for her, so as soon as she turns 65 she enrolls in Medicare Parts A and B. She has several medical conditions, including asthma. Her current medical policy is creditable, so one month after beginning Medicare she goes off her husband's policy and buys a Medigap policy. She is able to get a Medigap plan that has no waiting periods or exclusions, even for her asthma.

- Larry Gerard had been healthy all his life. He has generally been covered by employer-funded health insurance, but no longer has it. He learns that he should enroll in Medicare when he turns 65, or penalties can result; so he signs up for Medicare Parts A and B. Since Larry feels he's healthy, he chooses not to purchase a Medigap plan. Two years later he develops prostate cancer, and his medical expenses rise sharply. He wants to buy a Medigap policy but is having a lot of trouble finding one.

GUARANTEED ISSUE RIGHTS

There are situations in which a person who didn't purchase a Medigap policy during the Medigap Open Enrollment Period is still allowed to buy a Medigap policy without medical underwriting. Medicare refers to this as **guaranteed issue rights**. It's saying that, under certain specific conditions, you are guaranteed the ability to purchase a Medigap policy at the base rate and without pre-existing condition exclusions. The most common situation involves termination of insurance that provided the same type of benefits as a Medigap plan, such as an employer-sponsored plan or a retiree plan. Losing a job that had good health insurance is a frequently encountered example. There are also a number of other special cases that confer guaranteed issue rights, such as your current Medigap insurance company going out of business or your relocating to a geographic area where your present Medigap plan isn't available.

Guaranteed issue rights may also apply if you try a Medicare Advantage plan and then decide you want to switch to Original Medicare and purchase a Medigap plan. Perhaps you started in a Medicare Advantage plan when you first enrolled in Medicare, but then decided that Original Medicare would be better for you. Alternatively, you could have started in Original Medicare, then tried Medicare Advantage, and then elected to switch back. However, guaranteed issue rights apply only if you've been in the Medicare Advantage plan *for one year or less*. Once you've been covered by a Medicare Advantage plan (or more than one plan) for more than a year, you are subject to medical underwriting if you later want a Medigap policy.

In all cases, to maintain guaranteed issue rights you must sign up for the new plan within 63 calendar days of the date the previous coverage ended. A complete list of all the special circumstances that are covered by the guaranteed issue rights regulations can be found on the Medicare website at:

http://www.medicare.gov/supplement-other-insurance/when-can-i-buy-medigap/guaranteed-issue-rights-scenarios.html

Buying a Medigap Policy

Since many insurance companies sell Medigap policies, they have to compete for your business. Medicare regulations determine which benefits are covered by any lettered plan. As a result, the actual insurance coverage will be identical for all Medigap policies of a particular letter. Every Plan C provides exactly the same coverage as any other Plan C; and any Plan F is exactly the same as any other Plan F. The insurance companies don't even get to decide whether a medical service that you receive should be covered—Medicare determines that. If Medicare considers a service medically necessary and pays its portion of the fee, then the Medigap insurance carrier must also pay its portion.

The differences between insurance carriers become important when they are using medical underwriting. As discussed above, applying for a Medigap policy during your open enrollment period significantly limits the impact of medical underwriting. At most, a pre-existing condition can be excluded from coverage for the first six months. Not so if you're applying outside of your Medigap Open Enrollment Period and don't qualify for guaranteed issue rights. In these situations, each insurance company can use whatever criteria it wishes in evaluating you. If you have some pre-existing medical problems, various companies may view these medical conditions differently.

In looking at Medigap policies, you will have to understand the "rating" methodology used by each company in establishing premiums. There are three methods:

1. Community-rated: Everyone in a given geographic area is charged the same premium regardless of age. Premiums do not increase as you get older (except for inflation and some adjustments).

2. Issue-age-rated: Your premium is determined by your age when you buy the policy and doesn't increase as you get older (except for inflation and some adjustments).

3. Attained-age-rated: Your premium is based on your age at the time you are paying the premium, lower initially when you're younger and increasing each year as you grow older.

In thinking about these three options it's clear that an attained-age-rated policy can be less expensive initially, since premiums will rise each year. Thus, what seems less expensive when you buy it can turn out to be far more expensive years later. Make sure you understand which methods are being used when you consider different policies. State laws sometimes regulate which rating method must be used.

SHOP, SHOP, SHOP

When making a "big ticket" purchase, most people will shop for it. They look for price, service, and reputation. Buying a Medigap policy isn't that different from buying a car or a large-screen TV. A Medigap policy certainly qualifies as a "big ticket" item. Depending on the plan, the geographic area, and the presence or absence of medical underwriting, your policy may cost several thousand dollars per year—and the cost goes on year after year after year. The moral: Shop, Shop, Shop. And start early.

How should you go about shopping for your policy? The first step is to find out which companies sell policies in your area and which specific lettered plans each company offers. In some locales, there may be only a few options to choose from; in others, multiple companies will offer policies. You can start by contacting your State Health Insurance Assistance Program (SHIP) for a current list of plans available in your geographic area. In many states you can obtain a table listing all the available plans, the companies writing each plan type, and the premiums charged by each company.

Alternatively, you can call Medicare or go to the Medicare website at www.medicare.gov/find-a-plan/questions/medigap-home.aspx. The page will say *Medigap Policy Search*. Enter your zip code and click *Continue*. A page entitled *View All Medigap Policies* will list all lettered Medigap policies available in your area.

⚠ **Unfortunately, the pricing information listed under** *Estimated Annual Cost* **in Medicare's listing of Medigap policies for your area is virtually useless. There's a single absurdly high cost listed for each lettered plan type, but no company-specific prices. You will have to make inquiries on pricing yourself.**

By clicking in the last column on the right you'll get a list of all companies that sell policies of a particular letter. You can select one at a time to get their addresses, websites, telephone numbers, and pricing methods and then contact each company to get prices for its offerings. You will probably be surprised at how much variation there is in the prices charged by different companies. Some may charge two to three times as much as others for exactly the same plan.

Also, don't assume that a more comprehensive plan will be more expensive than a more basic one. I have seen examples of Plan F from one company being substantially less expensive than Plan A from another. That's hard to believe, I know, but it's true. The Cadillac of plans from one company was less costly than the Chevy from another! When I was looking at some plan prices recently, I was surprised to notice that one company was charging only $1 more per month for Plan F than for Plan C. You got Part B Excess Coverage, which pays for non-participating doctors, for a buck a month. Incredible!

> **THE POLICY THAT LOOKS LIKE YOUR BEST OPTION MAY NOT TURN OUT TO BE THE CHEAPEST OR EVEN AVAILABLE AT ALL.**

Some companies offer discounts on their regular rates based on gender or lifestyle (e.g., nonsmokers may pay less). Even though Original Medicare policies are always individual policies, some Medigap insurers will give discounts if both members of a couple insure with them.

The insurance companies writing Medigap policies can also compete by adding extra perks to their programs. Some provide toll-free numbers where you can get medical advice from registered nurses on a 24-hour basis. Some offer discounts on hearing aids. Free or discounted gym memberships may be included as well.

A MUCH SIMPLER WAY: USING AN INSURANCE AGENT

If researching Medigap plans sounds like a lot of work, it is. Another option is to seek out an insurance agent who sells Medigap policies. Some may work in general insurance agencies that deal with all types of insurance, including auto, homeowner's, and life insurance; others may specialize in the area of medical/life/long-term-care insurance. Agents receive commissions from the insurance companies, so you pay nothing extra. A good insurance agent will be familiar with the plans available in your state and the special regulations that your state laws impose. She can research various options for you and lay out different policies for you to choose from. Ideally, data on various plans from different companies will be presented in a table that makes comparisons easier. You'll be able to view on one sheet the different plans and their costs. Often the most advantageous choices will become readily apparent.

An agent's expertise may be especially helpful if you will have to undergo medical underwriting, since you may need to apply to several companies. You should know that an agent must be registered with each insurance company she represents, so any given agent may not be able to sell you a policy from every company. If you're having difficulty finding a policy, you might have to talk to more than one agent.

> **Final advice on choosing a Medigap policy:** Personally, I believe dealing with an insurance agent you trust is preferable to contacting each individual insurance carrier and trying to compare them on your own. It costs you nothing extra, will definitely save you time, and may well save you money. Incidentally, once you've read this chapter, any agent you talk to will be absolutely blown away by how much you know about Medigap plans!

If You're Considering Not Buying a Medigap Policy...

If, after reading this discussion of Medigap policies and thinking about your options, you decide that a Medigap policy is simply too expensive, think it through again and consider the following: A lengthy illness can be extremely costly, and Medicare cost sharing can result in out-of-pocket expenses of $10,000, $25,000, or more. Inability to pay large medical expenses is a major cause of bankruptcy in this country. Living with no Medigap plan in place is risky. A high-deductible Plan F can frequently be obtained quite reasonably, sometimes as low as $35 per month. Your maximum cost sharing exposure with a high-deductible Plan F is $2,140. In other words, for a modest monthly premium you can minimize the likelihood of ruinous medical bills.

Never forget the future. The Medigap policy you buy now may well be the policy you have for an indefinite period.

You are not guaranteed the right to change policies or insurance companies. If your health deteriorates, it is unlikely that a new insurance carrier will accept you at any reasonable cost, but the old one must keep you in your existing policy. As long as you continue to pay the premiums, your policy will remain in effect. Depending on your specific circumstances, failing to purchase a Medigap policy during your Medigap Open Enrollment Period may prevent you from ever being able to get a reasonable one. Think carefully about the choices you make now.

The Future of Medigap

You should also be aware that the entire concept of supplemental Medicare insurance has been coming under fire. Critics contend that having total coverage (as provided by the more comprehensive plans) leads to wasteful overutilization of medical services, thereby driving up overall government expenditures for Medicare. Studies have shown that Medicare pays out 25% more for enrollees who have Medigap policies than for those who don't.[1] If all recipients had to pay something for every medical service they received, the reasoning goes, they would look for less expensive options and seek fewer services. Proposals have included combining Medicare Parts A and B and instituting a single large (perhaps $500) annual deductible that couldn't be covered by Medigap. President Obama has proposed adding a surcharge (that would go to CMS) for newly purchased Medigap policies that provide first-dollar coverage (like C and F). Exactly what changes to Medigap will be enacted is speculative at present. In the past, individuals with existing Medigap policies have been guaranteed the right to keep them even after rule changes; for legal reasons it's likely this would pertain in the future—all the more reason to buy a Medigap policy as soon as you can.

Key Points for Medigap

- Medigap policies are specifically designed to provide insurance covering cost sharing in Medicare Parts A and B.

- Sold by private insurance companies under strict Medicare guidelines—only standardized Medigap policies.

- Lettered policies include different combinations of Medigap benefits.

---

[1] Jaffee, Susan "Officials Looking to Cut Federal Spending Eye Medigap Policies," Kaiser Health News Nov 2, 2011 http://www.kaiserhealthnews.org/Stories/2011/November/ss/Medigap-and-federal-policies.aspx

- Decide which Medigap benefits are important to you and shop aggressively; prices for identical policies can vary tremendously.

- A more comprehensive policy from one company may be less expensive than an inferior policy from another.

- Buy during the Medigap Open Enrollment Period to limit medical underwriting.

- Understand the importance of medical underwriting if you're beyond the Medigap Open Enrollment Period.

- Consider a high-deductible Plan F if you feel most plans are too costly; this plan type may also be the best deal for those of you who can afford other plans.

- Using an insurance agent can make the process much easier, will cost you nothing, and may actually save you money.

Bottom-Line Recommendations:

- Think very carefully before opting not to buy a Medigap policy. It's a decision that could cost you thousands of dollars in the future.

- Buy a Medigap policy during the Medigap Open Enrollment Period or you could be rejected by insurers, charged a much higher premium rate, or have pre-existing conditions excluded.

- Shop around. Better coverage is not always more expensive coverage.

Chapter 5

Medicare Part D—Medicare Drug Plans

"This isn't Part C? It should be. C for Confusing. On the other hand, maybe Part D really is a good name—D for Donut Hole."

Medicare Part D (think "D for Drugs") is the final component of Original Medicare, although it was not part of the program as initially created. For most of the time that Medicare has been in existence, no medication coverage was available. Some seniors had drug benefits from retiree plans, and some Medigap policies included medications. (These were Plans E, H, I, and J, which ceased to be available with the advent of Medicare Part D.) However, the majority of Medicare recipients were on their own when it came to paying for their drugs. As medications became more numerous, more sophisticated, and more expensive, the absence of drug coverage became a progressively greater financial burden for seniors.

In 2006, Congress finally added a prescription drug benefit: Medicare Part D. The debate over this plan was contentious and rancorous. The pharmaceutical industry lobbied aggressively against it, afraid that the buying power of a large government program would lower prices. Some congressmen contended the bill was too costly and would add to "big government," while others felt it didn't go nearly far enough. The final legislation—the result of major compromises--was a breakthrough in benefits for seniors, but it was far from a perfect bill. In particular, the notorious "donut hole" was included. Since then, refinements have been enacted, and the program continues to evolve—mostly for the better.

What's Included in Part D Plans?

Medicare Part D covers only *prescription* medications. No matter how important you feel an over-the-counter drug may be for your health, Medicare drug plans won't pay for it. This has become a problem for some seniors, since several widely used medications that formerly required prescriptions have become nonprescription. Some antihistamines used for allergies are notable examples. Also:

- Medications given to hospital inpatients are covered by Medicare Part A, not Part D.

- Certain medicines administered in doctors' offices and other outpatient settings, most notably cancer chemotherapy drugs, are covered under Medicare Part B, not Part D.

- Most prescriptions you fill at a pharmacy, including mail-order pharmacies, do fall under Part D. However, Medicare's rules specifically exclude certain medications, and plans generally don't cover all available drugs.

Who Qualifies for Medicare Part D?

Anyone who is eligible for Medicare Part A or Medicare Part B also qualifies for Medicare drug coverage. Even though Part D plans are run by private insurance companies, no one can be turned down, and there can be no medical underwriting. Period. Those who participate in Original Medicare obtain their benefits by enrolling in separate Part D drug plans, while those in most Medicare Advantage programs now receive drug coverage as part of the plans' benefits packages. If a particular Medicare Advantage plan doesn't include medications, the enrollee can purchase a separate Part D plan that's the same as those for Original Medicare recipients

Should I Sign Up?

A Medicare prescription drug plan definitely costs money, sometimes a substantial amount. As a result, if you have other insurance that provides drug coverage, you might want to defer starting Medicare Part D. In many cases, a drug benefit that's part of an employer-sponsored insurance plan or retiree benefit plan is better and cheaper than Part D. Medicare regulations do allow you to do this, irrespective of the source of that insurance. However, your alternative drug plan must provide creditable coverage, which means that Medicare considers it at least as good as Part D. Your insurance carrier will provide you with documentation that the coverage is indeed creditable.

Medicare Part D has an **Initial Enrollment Period,** which, for most of you, is the seven-month period that includes the three months before your 65th birthday, the month of your 65th birthday, and the subsequent three months. This is exactly the same Initial Enrollment Period you learned about earlier for Medicare Parts A and B.

There are also **Special Enrollment Periods**. Let's say you had creditable coverage for a year or two and then lost it because you stopped working. Or perhaps your former employer discontinued your retiree benefit plan. In such situations, you qualify for a Special Enrollment Period and can join Medicare Part D without penalty.

Part D Late Enrollment Penalties

⚠️ **Failure to enroll in a Medicare Part D plan in a timely manner can result in lifelong penalties. Don't get trapped because you feel you don't need a drug plan.**

What happens if you simply don't want to enroll in a Medicare Part D plan? Perhaps you take no medications at all, or you take a few and they don't cost very much. You feel the plans are simply too expensive for your needs. Medicare cannot force you to join, but you are taking a risk. First off, your health could change at any time. Who can predict the future? If you suddenly develop a severe illness, your drug bills could go from almost nothing to hundreds or even thousands of dollars a month overnight. At that point, you wouldn't be able to get a Medicare Part D plan until the next **Open Enrollment Period,** which occurs yearly between October 15th and December 7th with coverage commencing on January 1st. You could go for many months without drug coverage.

Second, if you don't enroll in a Medicare Part D plan during an Initial or Special Enrollment Period, substantial penalties will kick in when you finally do sign up. *You will pay an additional amount on your monthly premium for as long as you participate (most likely for the rest of your life). Specifically, there is a 1% premium penalty for each month that you delay enrolling in Medicare Part D.* Let's say you became Part D eligible at age 65 but chose not to sign up for three years. Now you're 68 and decide you need Part D benefits. You've delayed for 36 months at 1% per month, which equals 36%. You will pay a penalty of 36% per month indefinitely.

Some of you might say, "No problem. I've heard that Part D premiums can vary considerably. I'll simply select a plan with a very low monthly premium, so the penalty won't be that bad." Not so fast. Medicare doesn't use *your* premium to calculate penalties. Rather, it uses what's called the "national base beneficiary premium," which changes every year. For 2014, the value is $32.42. Thus, in the above example, your penalty would be 36% of $32.42, or $11.67 every month. These penalties can add up. If you feel you don't really want a Medicare Part D plan but wish to avoid these penalties in the future, one strategy is to select the least expensive plan you can find for now. You can change plans later as your medication needs evolve.

Changing Plans

Did I just say that you could join one plan and then change plans later? Yes, I did. One important feature of Medicare Part D is that *you can switch plans every year without penalty.* If you're unhappy with your plan for any reason, you can drop the plan and enroll in another. If you've happy with it but you develop new health problems that require different medications, you can change for that reason too. Once a year, during the period October 15th to December 7th, you are free to leave a plan, enroll in a plan, or change plans; your new plan will become effective on January 1st. If you move to a new plan, you won't even need to inform your previous one—your coverage in the old plan will automatically end when the new one begins.

You can switch to what's called a 5-star Medicare Prescription Drug Plan at any point during the year. The star ratings are based on a number of criteria established by Medicare (discussed more fully later). It's very difficult to get five stars, and many good plans can't get them—it's hard to please all the people all the time. You may not be able to find one in your area.

Moving out of your plan's service area is another permissible reason to change plans in mid-year. All Medicare Part D plans are specific to a particular locality, and you don't necessarily have to move very far to leave your plan's service area. In this situation, you can enroll in a plan in your new area without penalty. Depending on the plan's structure, you may have a new deductible. It's your responsibility to contact Medicare when you move and need to find a new plan.

How Does a Medicare Part D Plan Work?

All Medicare Part D plans are sponsored and administered by private insurance companies under specific Medicare guidelines. In this respect, they are similar to the Medigap policies discussed in the previous chapter. Where they differ is that, while all Medigap policies of a given letter (A, C, F, etc.) are identical, Part D drug plans vary tremendously.[2] Medicare has established rules under which all plans must operate, but there is wide latitude regarding how plans may structure their charges and benefits. For example:

- Medicare determines the range of monthly premiums that can be charged by a plan, but insurers can set the premiums wherever they want within that range.

- Medicare dictates the maximum annual deductible, but any given plan can use that amount, a lesser amount, or no deductible at all.

- Medicare has a list of drugs that are not covered by Medicare Part D and also specifies certain drugs that must be covered. Additionally, Medicare requires that at least two separate medications be available in every drug category (see the box on page 71). But each company can decide which specific drugs will be included in its plan and how much each will cost.

Within these parameters, each insurance carrier can create its own Part D plans using varying combinations of premiums, deductibles, copays, and coinsurance. The number of possible variations is staggering. As a result, Medicare Part D plans are complicated—absurdly complicated. These plans are definitely not "one size fits all." There are countless available options. Cost sharing can be

---

[2] Another area where Medigap and Part D differ is that a Medigap policy is a contract between an individual and an insurance company, and the purchaser pays 100% of the cost of the policy, whereas Medicare Part D policies are heavily subsidized by CMS. The total amount that Medicare recipients pay for premiums and cost sharing does not come close to the cost of running Medicare Part D. In fact, the federal government pays approximately 75% of the overall expense of supplying Part D medications.

structured in many ways. Drugs available in some plans may not be available in others. The price of a particular medication can vary from plan to plan; additionally, the cost of a drug will change as you move through sequential payment stages (including the donut hole) characteristic of all Part D plans.

These concepts and options can be baffling. There is no simple way to explain Medicare Part D; but I'm going to try. If you're not familiar with the terms that insurers use for medication coverage, start your Medicare Part D 101 course with the Important Drug Definitions box below. Then bear with me to the end and, hopefully, it will finally become clear. Here goes.

Important Drug Definitions

Some of the following terms may already be familiar to you from previous experiences with medical insurance, but they're critical to understanding these plans.

Brand-name drug—A brand-name drug is a medication that is still covered by a U.S. patent. As a result, it can be made and sold by only one pharmaceutical company—the company that developed it or that licensed it from the developer. The company controls the price, so these medications tend to be the most expensive. The name of a brand-name drug starts with a capital letter (e.g., Lipitor).

Generic drug—A generic drug is a medication that is no longer under patent protection. As a result, it can be manufactured and sold by many drug companies. Since there is competition among these companies, prices tend to be lower. The name of a generic drug will often start with a small letter (e.g., atorvastatin, which is generic Lipitor).

Formulary—A formulary is the complete list of all drugs covered by a particular drug plan. Most formularies contain both brand-name and generic drugs. If a particular drug is not included in a plan's formulary, there is generally no coverage whatever for that drug. The exact composition of any formulary is determined by the individual insurance company managing the plan.

Tier—The medications in any given formulary are divided into what are called "tiers," which are levels of coverage. Most Medicare Part D programs have between three and five tiers that contain all the drugs in their formularies. Tier 1 drugs tend to have the lowest cost to you, while the higher tiers cost the most. Typically, tier 1 will contain the plan's basic generic drugs. Tier 2 often has nonpreferred generics or preferred brand-name drugs, which are brand-name medications for which the plan has negotiated special prices. The highest tiers contain other brand-name drugs and specialty drugs.

Category—Drugs in the same category are those that treat a specific disease by a particular mechanism. For example, ACE inhibitors (full name *angiotensin converting enzyme inhibitors*), a class of drug commonly used to treat high blood pressure, constitute one category. Drugs that treat high blood pressure by a different specific mechanism, such as beta blockers, would constitute a second category.

The Structure of a Medicare Part D Plan

How is a Medicare Part D Plan constructed? Essentially, each plan decides which drugs it will cover and how you will pay for them. Here are the building blocks that make up all Medicare Part D plans:

PREMIUMS

- Every Part D plan has a **monthly premium**. This is the amount you pay each month simply to be a member of the plan. You pay it whether you fill any prescriptions or not.

- Individuals with higher incomes pay an additional monthly premium for Part D coverage. It's based on modified adjusted gross income (MAGI) and is analogous to the additional premiums paid by higher-income recipients for Medicare Part B. Approximately 5% of enrollees must pay it. The additional income-related premiums for 2014 are shown in the table below. You pay your plan's monthly premium directly to the insurance company underwriting the plan. However, any income-related additional premium goes directly to CMS, either as a deduction from your monthly Social Security payment or, if you are not yet receiving Social Security benefits, as a check or bank debit.

Part D Additional Premiums by Income for 2014

If your modified adjusted gross income in 2012 was:		You Pay in 2014
File individual tax return	File joint tax return	
$85,000 or less	$170,000 or less	None
above $85,000 up to $107,000	above $170,000 up to $214,000	$12.10
above $107,000 up to $160,000	above $214,000 up to $320,000	$31.10
above $160,000 up to $214,000	above $320,000 up to $428,000	$50.20
above $214,000	above $428,000	$69.30

COST SHARING

- A plan may have an **annual deductible**, which is the amount you must pay for covered medications before the plan pays anything. Medicare sets a maximum allowable annual deductible-- currently $310. Many plans charge much less than $310, and some impose no annual deductible at all.

- **Copays** and **coinsurance** are important components of all Part D plans. They can be used in various combinations. In a typical situation, there is a low copay for tier 1 drugs, a higher copay for tier 2 drugs, and much higher ones for tiers 3 and above. The highest tier often utilizes coinsurance instead; that is, for very expensive drugs you pay a percentage of the cost rather than a fixed copay. Some plans use coinsurance for all drugs. In this scenario, you pay a percentage of the cost of all medications in all tiers.

FORMULARIES AND TIERS

- The specific constellation of medications chosen for inclusion in any plan's formulary is up to the plan sponsor. As mentioned earlier, Medicare requires at least two choices in any drug category, but those two may represent only a small fraction of available drugs. (For example, there are about ten different ACE inhibitors—discussed in the box on Important Drug Definitions—currently marketed in the United States. A plan may choose to make many of them available, or could include only two.) Some plans have far more comprehensive formularies than others.

- The number of tiers and how they are defined are totally up to the plan. Four tiers and five tiers are common. Additionally, which drugs are allocated to each tier is solely at the discretion of the plan. As a rule, cost sharing parameters are set up to encourage you to use tier 1 drugs by making them substantially less expensive than those in higher tiers.

- For certain medical conditions, Medicare requires that substantially all available drugs be included in every formulary. These include chemotherapy drugs (cancer treatments), anticonvulsants (seizure drugs), antidepressants, antipsychotics, HIV/AIDS drugs, and immunosuppressive agents (for autoimmune disorders and organ transplants).

- Medicare also prohibits coverage for certain drugs. These include barbiturates (sedatives), benzodiazepines (like Valium); prescription vitamins; and drugs to treat weight gain, weight loss (except in AIDS patients), hair growth, infertility, and erectile dysfunction. As noted earlier, all over-the-counter drugs are similarly excluded. A plan can choose to pay for any of these or offer discounts for them, but Medicare will not pay any portion of the cost.

RESTRICTIONS

- Some drugs may be included in a formulary but carry with them certain restrictions. A specific medication may require **prior authorization,** whereby your doctor must file a specific request with the plan before prescribing the drug. The plan may or may not approve the request. For other drugs, **quantity limits** may be imposed; only a set number of pills will be allowed during a given time period. **Step therapy** requires that a cheaper drug (usually a generic or preferred brand-name drug) be tried prior to authorizing a more expensive one.

- Many plans restrict where you can fill your prescriptions. Some require you to use only specific pharmacies, while others lower your cost sharing if you choose preferred pharmacies. For some plans the pharmacy choices are extensive; for others less so. Most plans allow you to use mail-order pharmacies and even encourage it. Especially when you order a three-month supply of a medication, utilizing mail-order may result in lower copays.

THE CONCEPT OF "FULL PRICE"

Every drug that is covered by a plan has a "full price," which is determined by what the plan pays for the drug. It will not be the same in all plans and can, in fact, vary considerably. Plans are able to negotiate prices with their drug suppliers, and you get the benefits of these reductions. The full price of any drug is important to you when you are still paying your deductible and when you enter the donut hole, which is discussed below. Also, they are extremely important in any plan where you always pay a percentage of full price (coinsurance) rather than fixed copays.

LOCATION

All Medicare Part D plans are specific to a particular geographic area. They are not necessarily available statewide and may encompass quite small areas. Available plans and costs can vary significantly from locality to locality.

Every Medicare Drug Plan has the following characteristics:

- A monthly premium

- Cost sharing that uses some combination of monthly premiums, an annual deductible, copays, and coinsurance

- A formulary that includes all drugs covered by the plan

- A tier system to group drugs that have similar cost sharing properties

- A full price for every drug in the formulary

- Certain restrictions, which may include prior authorizations, quantity limits, and step therapy

How Medicare Regulates Part D Plan Charges

As you can now see, the number of ways in which plans can vary is almost infinite. Why, then, shouldn't you just select a plan that has the lowest possible premium, no deductible, a huge formulary, and the lowest copays? Because it doesn't exist. If a plan is low cost in one area, it will be higher in others. Medicare has established that all plans must, in aggregate, cover 75% of the medication costs of the individuals in the plan. This does *not* mean 75% of each person's costs. Rather, total outlays of the plan must be "actuarially equivalent" to 75% of the total drug costs of all its Plan D policy holders. Some of you will benefit more than others, depending on what medications you use, what tiers contain your drugs, and how clever you were in selecting a plan. The best choice for you will be the one with the optimum combination of covered drugs and costs for your particular medical needs. Later on, I'll discuss how to choose.

The Infamous Donut Hole

Undoubtedly the most enigmatic and distressing component of Medicare Part D is the donut hole, which is not its real name. It's officially called the **coverage gap.** This gap resulted from the congressional negotiations that led to Part D's creation in 2006. Some legislators feared that Medicare's expenditures for drugs would become far too great, so they wanted a cap placed on the amount that would be covered for each recipient. Others noted that one of the great tragedies of our medical system was that huge medication costs could impoverish seniors and their families. The compromise resulted in a program that paid benefits up to a certain level and then stopped, only to begin again at a higher level to cover catastrophic situations. The coverage gap (the donut hole) was the zone where the plan paid nothing toward drug costs. This concept is unique to Medicare Part D. Do you know of any other type of insurance that has a hole in the middle?

From a practical perspective, here's how it works.

- The Medicare Part D plan pays its portion of drug costs until the total amount expended in a given year reaches $2,850. This total includes amounts paid out by the plan plus all deductibles, copays, and coinsurance paid by you. It specifically does NOT include your monthly premiums.

- Once this ceiling of $2,850 is reached, you enter the coverage gap--you're in the donut hole! At this point, the amount you pay is determined by the full price of each drug and is substantially higher.

- Once your "out-of pocket expenditures" total $4,550, you leave the coverage gap and qualify for catastrophic coverage.

What exactly are your costs when you're in the donut hole? When Medicare Part D was first created, you had to pay 100% of full price. More recently, through agreements with the pharmaceutical industry and as part of the Affordable Care Act (ObamaCare), there are now subsidies for drug costs in the donut hole. In 2014:

- For any generic drug, you pay 72% of the plan's cost for the drug.

- For any brand-name drug, you pay 47.5% of the plan's cost, with the pharmaceutical industry picking up the remaining 52.5%.

- The proportion you pay will decrease progressively until 2020, at which time you will pay 25% for all drug types. The donut hole will have essentially disappeared.

As noted above, you exit the coverage gap when all your "out-of-pocket expenditures" reach $4,550. How does Medicare define this very important $4,550 limit?

- First, it includes all deductibles, copays, and coinsurance paid by you prior to reaching the coverage gap. Second, it includes everything you paid for generic and brand-name drugs while in the coverage gap. Third, it includes the portion kicked in by the pharmaceutical companies for your brand-name drug while in the coverage gap.

- Your costs for drugs that were not on your plan's formulary and for drugs excluded by Medicare don't count.

"Out-of-pocket expenditures" is NOT the same as "total cost," which is used to determine when you enter the coverage gap. "Total cost" includes amounts paid by the plan, whereas "out-of-pocket expenditures" does not. This may seem ridiculous, but it's the way the donut hole was designed. To repeat, you enter the donut hole when "total costs" paid by you and the plan reach $2,850, but you exit when your "out-of-pocket expenditures" (including the pharmaceutical industry contributions) reach $4,550.

Once this $4,550 threshold has been reached, you're out of the coverage gap and qualify for catastrophic coverage, whereby you pay very small copays or coinsurance for all your drugs. Medicare specifies standard catastrophic cost sharing rules that pertain to all Part D plans. You pay either the copay determined by Medicare or 5% of the cost of the drug, whichever is greater.

Drug Payment Stages

You are not alone if you find the cost structure of Part D incomprehensible. There is another way to look at it, which some people find easier: Think of your Part D costs as having four distinct payment stages that you move through sequentially.

- Stage 1—Yearly deductible: During this period you pay "full price" for all medications until your deductible has been met. If your plan requires no deductible, you skip this first stage.

- Stage 2—Initial coverage: Once you've fulfilled your deductible, you pay only the copay or coinsurance for each prescription medication as specified by the tier structure of your plan. You remain in this stage until "total drug costs" (annual deductible, coinsurance and copays paid by you, and expenditures paid by the plan) reach $2,850.

- Stage 3—Coverage gap (donut hole): Once total costs exceed $2,850, you pay 72% of the plan's cost for any generic drugs in the plan's formulary and approximately 47.5% for any brand-name drugs in that formulary. You remain in this stage until your total "out-of pocket costs" (as defined earlier) reach $4,550.

- Stage 4—Catastrophic coverage: Once you leave the coverage gap (the donut hole), your drug expenses drop sharply. In this final stage, cost sharing expenses are determined by Medicare's rules. You pay only the standard catastrophic copay or 5% of the cost of any drug, whichever is greater.

At the end of the calendar year, the stages start all over again. It doesn't matter where you were on December 31st; on January 1st you'll be right back at the beginning of the cycle.

⚠️ **No matter what stage you're in, you must continue to pay the monthly premiums—both to your plan and to CMS if your income so dictates.**

Many people never totally understand how these stages really work until they get personally involved with their own medication expenses. Once you have a Part D plan, you will receive a monthly statement called an **explanation of benefits** from your Part D insurance carrier. It will list all the prescriptions you've filled during the month, along with how much you and the insurance company paid for them. Additionally, it will indicate what your "total expenditures" were for the month and year to date, along with information about what stage you're presently in and how much extra spending will move you to the next stage. We'll look at a Part D explanation of benefits in Chapter 11, "Using Your Medicare Wisely."

Enrolling in a Medicare Part D Plan

Signing up for a Medicare Part D Plan is quite simple. You can enroll in any plan through Medicare, either online at www.medicare.gov or on the phone at 1-800-MEDICARE. Alternatively, you can enroll through the plan itself. You can use the plan's website, fill out a paper application, or apply on the phone. The applications are easy to complete. Remember, a Medicare Part D plan must accept anyone who applies for it. Medical underwriting never applies.

⚠ You cannot legally be enrolled in a Medicare drug plan if the company calls <u>you</u> on the phone. Indeed, Part D plan representatives are forbidden from soliciting your business in that way. They can send you literature in the mail, but any telephone call must be initiated by you. This protection was put into place by CMS to eliminate high-pressure sales tactics by plan representatives. Do not buy a plan from anyone who has made an unsolicited telephone call to you.

Researching Part D Plans

The hard part is *selecting* the right plan for your needs. Fortunately, your choice is not permanent. As mentioned earlier, you can change plans once a year. Nevertheless, you will have the plan for a full year, so it's advisable to choose wisely from the start. Outlines of three typical plans are depicted in the table below. These are theoretical examples, but they approximate the kinds of options you'll encounter in the real world.

Comparison of Three Typical Part D Plans

Plan	Monthly Premium	Deductible	Copay (1-Month Supply)
X	$40	$50	Tier 1 - $4
			Tier 2 - $15
			Tier 3 - $40
			Tier 4 - $90
			Tier 5 – 35% coinsurance
Y	$25	$310	25% coinsurance for all drugs

Plan	Monthly Premium	Deductible	Copay (1-Month Supply)
Z	$85	None	Tier 1 - $0
			Tier 2 - $10
			Tier 3 - $ 85
			Tier 4 – 30% coinsurance

In looking at these examples, you'll note significant variations among them. For a person who takes no medications and wants the absolute cheapest way to enroll in a Medicare drug plan (possibly to avoid penalties later on), Plan Y might be a reasonable choice. It has a low monthly premium, and the high deductible is not important if you take little medication; but if you take lots of drugs, the 25% coinsurance could rapidly become prohibitively expensive. Plans X and Z are typical Part D programs that could work well for those taking moderate amounts of medication. Beyond that, though, the table really doesn't help much. Why? Because it doesn't tell us which drugs are on each formulary and which of them are located in each tier. In other words, it tells us nothing about how each plan deals with specific medications—*your medications*.

To make a rational decision regarding which plan is best for you, you need the ability to analyze your total cost given the exact drugs you take. Trying to do this by hand would be a daunting task. In any given locality, there may be 30, 40, or even 50 available plans to choose from. Computers, however, are very good at making lots of calculations rapidly. Fortunately, Medicare provides you with a truly excellent tool to help. It's called the **Medicare Plan Finder**, and it's available for you to use at www.medicare.gov. You will find it remarkably user friendly. If you're not comfortable with online programs, get someone to help you. Perhaps you have a friend who's really adept at using the internet. Many senior centers have people available to provide assistance.

Specific instructions for using this online tool most effectively are provided in **Appendix B**. Step-by-step directions will guide you through the program and suggest how to answer questions to get the information you need to compare available plans. Take the time to explore this tool using the recommendations in **Appendix B** as your guide.

⚠ Although the *Medicare Plan Finder* can help you make the choice that's best for you <u>right now,</u> keep in mind that there's always a chance your needs will change and the plan in which you've enrolled will no longer be the best deal. New medical problems could result in your needing an entirely different set of medications, possibly expensive ones. Perhaps you take only generic drugs now, but all of a sudden you require several sophisticated brand-name medications with no generic alternatives. Most important, your new drugs could easily push you into the dreaded donut hole. If you were to put your new drug list into the *Medicare Plan Finder*, the plan you originally selected might no longer be the most favorable.

Though you clearly cannot foresee what medication changes might be needed in the future, you should consider at least asking your doctors if they anticipate any major modifications of your drug regimens.

Fortunately, should significant increases in your drugs outlays occur, you can change plans next year and hopefully limit these unanticipated extra costs.

Making Your Decision

Once you've spent some time with the *Medicare Plan Finder*, you'll probably have a pretty good idea of which plans appear to be best for you. From a cost perspective, certain plans will clearly stand out. However, there are factors beyond present cost that you should consider. An important one is the reputation of the insurance company running the plan. Having been a practicing physician for over 30 years, I can tell you with assurance that there are tremendous differences among insurance carriers. Some are easy to deal with and tend to approve requests expeditiously. Some can be extremely oppositional whenever a specific authorization is needed. We've had instances when it was virtually impossible to reach anyone on the phone. My staff members would spend long periods on hold or, once they did get through, end up being transferred from person to person. It was very clear that our call was *not* very important to them, notwithstanding the recorded statements that greeted us. Remember that all drugs are not automatically approved—some need prior authorization, while some will have quantity limitations and others are subject to step therapy rules. In these situations, your doctors will need to contact your Plan D carrier. Creating extra work and problems for your doctor and staff can strain a patient-doctor relationship, even if it's not your fault.

How can you avoid ending up with a nightmarish insurance company? Help is available.

THE STAR RATING SYSTEM

How can you know which insurance carriers will be the easiest for you and your doctors to deal with? You can't know for sure, but reputations can certainly be helpful. Toward this end, Medicare has created a system which uses a 5-star scale for rating plans. If you went through using the *Medicare Plan Finder* as outlined in Appendix B, you undoubtedly noted the star ratings listed for each plan. In determining the star ratings, Medicare uses 17 factors that include quality of customer service, how appeals are handled, complaints against the plan, how many members leave the plan, problems that Medicare discovers, and pricing considerations. Data is obtained from Medicare's own inquiries and from member satisfaction surveys.

⚠ **The star ratings you see on the website will not be the same as the star ratings you'll find in the plan listings in the booklet *Medicare and You*. The ratings on the website include all 17 factors noted above, while those in the booklet are based on patient satisfaction surveys. The website ratings will almost invariably be lower. You'll see very few 4- and 5-star ratings there. Three and 3 1/2 stars are OK. Be cautious of ratings below that. You'll definitely see 5-star ratings in *Medicare and You*. If a company tells you that it is 4- or 5-star rated, make sure you know which rating the representative is talking about. Check for yourself online in the *Medicare Plan Finder*.**

AN EASIER WAY: USING AN INSURANCE AGENT

As with choosing a Medigap plan, one of the best methods for selecting a drug plan may be to consult an insurance agent. A knowledgeable agent can help you examine the various plan options and assist you in using the website. Some will actually do the online analysis for you and create printed plan comparisons using your particular medication list. Additionally, agents who do a lot of work with Medicare Part D plans can provide you with knowledge gained from the experiences of their other clients. They often have insights into which companies have proven easiest to deal with and which have not. This type of personal, local information can be invaluable. Any agent who sells Medicare Part D plans must be licensed by the state and must be registered with each insurance company whose plans he sells. The insurance companies require agents to take special training courses and sometimes exams so that they are familiar with the products offered. As with Medigap policies, commissions are paid by the insurance companies; there is no cost to you for using an insurance agent.

If you employ the services of an agent, make sure you go to someone you know, or someone who was recommended by someone you trust. Medicare Part D policies are profitable for the companies that underwrite them. As such, salesmen can sometimes be quite aggressive in promoting them. They may represent only one company and push that carrier's particular products. I prefer agents who can sell you policies from many different insurance companies, since they can show you a wide variety of options.

You will probably get lots of literature in the mail from multiple sources. As mentioned earlier, Medicare regulations state that no agent or representative of any Part D plan can solicit you on the telephone or by coming to your door, only by mail. Once you contact them, however, you may be subject to a hard sell. Make sure you know with whom you're dealing. If anyone attempts to contact you by phone or in person, and you haven't previously requested information from that company, report the incident to Medicare (at 1-800-MEDICARE).

What is the *Extra Help* Program?

For low-income individuals, Medicare provides a program called *Extra Help* that reduces drug costs. Specific limitations on annual income and financial resources apply. Recipients of full Medicaid and certain other programs automatically qualify; others must apply through Social Security and show evidence of their financial situations. More information about the requirements and benefits of the *Extra Help* program are available in *Medicare and You*, on the Medicare.gov website, or by calling Social Security at 1-800-772-1213. For those who don't qualify for *Extra Help* but have burdensome medication costs, additional resources are available in some states. These can be explored by contacting the local State Health Insurance Assistance Program (SHIP).

Key Points for Medicare Part D
(Medicare Drug Plans)

- Medicare Part D covers outpatient prescriptions you fill at a pharmacy or receive by mail order.

- Plans are run by private insurance companies under Medicare guidelines.

- A monthly premium is paid to the insurance company sponsoring the plan. As with Part B, those with higher MAGI pay more; the additional amounts go to CMS.

- Enroll during the Initial Enrollment Period or a Special Enrollment Period (available if you have creditable alternative drug coverage) without penalty.

- Failure to enroll at the proper times will result in a lifelong penalty of 1% per month for every month you delay enrolling.

- You can change plans yearly without penalty.

- Plans can be structured to include various combinations of premiums, deductibles, copays, and coinsurance.

- Each plan establishes a formulary that includes all covered drugs.

- Drugs are assigned to tiers, which are levels of coverage, with generics in the lowest tiers and specialty drugs in the highest ones.

- Cost of a particular drug varies by stage: Full price during the annual deductible stage, a copay or coinsurance based on tier during the initial coverage stage, a modified full price during the coverage gap (donut hole), and a much lower amount during the catastrophic stage.

- Entering and leaving the coverage gap is complicated; coverage gap being phased out by 2020.

- Evaluating various plans is so complicated that the use of an Internet-based tool called the *Medicare Plan Finder* is necessary.

- **Use of an insurance agent can make choosing a plan simpler and may save you money.**

Bottom-Line Recommendations:

- Sign up during the designated enrollment periods to avoid penalties that could last for the rest of your life.

- Use the *Medicare Plan Finder* and/or a known insurance agent to help you compare plans by cost and the star ratings that rank companies according to other quality factors.

- Be prepared to change plans during the annual Open Enrollment Period (October 15th through December 7th), because the plan that's best now might no longer be the best one for you as time goes on.

Chapter 6

Medicare Part C—Medicare Advantage Plans

"Part A, Part B, Part D ... Plan A, Plan F, Plan N. Way too much to figure out. I want one insurance plan with one card— just like I used to have."

The last few chapters have gone over what it takes to develop a complete, comprehensive insurance program for any senior who qualifies for Medicare. Under Original Medicare, you'll have Medicare Parts A and B for inpatient care, doctors, and laboratories, plus a Medigap policy to help with Medicare's cost sharing requirements. Your Medicare Part D plan will add drug coverage. But isn't it very cumbersome to have all these separate plans? In many ways it is. You will certainly have several separate medical insurance cards. Every time you go to a hospital, doctor, or laboratory, you'll have to present both your Medicare card and your Medigap card. If you forget either card when you seek medical services, you'll very rapidly start getting bills from your providers. And you'll have to present an entirely different card for medications.

Isn't there a way to get all your coverage under one integrated plan? Yes. You can get comprehensive coverage without having to pay for a Medigap plan by opting for Medicare Part C, better known as Medicare Advantage. You'll also see the term Medicare Health Plan, especially on the Medicare website. All three names mean basically the same thing.

> MEDICARE PART C = MEDICARE ADVANTAGE = MEDICARE HEALTH PLAN

What Exactly Is a Medicare Advantage Plan?

Medicare Advantage (MA) plans are insurance programs run by private insurance companies under specific Medicare guidelines. They must cover essentially the same services as Original Medicare, but not necessarily in the same way. For each individual enrolled in a Medicare

Advantage plan, Medicare pays the plan a fixed dollar amount per month to provide care for that person. This amount is based on Medicare's average monthly expenditures for Original Medicare enrollees in a given geographic area. There are also some adjustments based on the specific medical problems of the individuals covered by a particular MA insurance carrier.

When you sign up for a Medicare Advantage plan, you are still a Medicare participant, but you don't have Original Medicare and you can't buy a Medigap policy. In recent years, drug coverage has also become integrated into most MA programs, so you probably won't need a separate Part D plan either. All your medical insurance coverage is supplied by the MA plan. Your medical care options and your cost sharing will both be determined by the rules and regulations of the specific MA plan you select, and these will differ significantly from Original Medicare.

Who Can Participate? When Can I Sign Up?

Any senior who qualifies for Medicare may choose to participate in a Medicare Advantage plan rather than Original Medicare.

⚠️ **The only exception to eligibility for Medicare Part C is patients with end-stage renal disease (kidney failure).**

All other seniors must be accepted by any Medicare Advantage plan they choose. Medical underwriting is not permissible, so pre-existing conditions make no difference. The fees that an MA plan charges must be the same for everyone who joins that plan.

You can join a Medicare Advantage plan when you first become eligible for Medicare during your Initial Enrollment Period. Alternatively, you can switch from Original Medicare to an MA plan or from one MA plan to another one during an annual Open Enrollment Period, which is October 15th to December 7th (the same period as for switching Medicare Part D Plans). Your new plan then takes effect on January 1st. You are allowed to change plans every year, if you're so inclined. If you move out of your plan's service area, you may switch to another one in your new home area at any time. You'll need to contact Medicare to tell them about your relocation. You may switch to a 5-star Medicare Advantage

Plan at any time during the year, provided that one is available in your area.

⚠ **When you switch plans during a plan year, you will still be responsible for new annual deductibles or premiums, even if you've already paid them in the old plan, so beware of switching mid-year.**

Managed Care: The Pros and Cons of Medicare Advantage Versus Original Medicare

Unlike Original Medicare, under which you can choose which providers to see and have the costs covered (as long as that doctor agrees to see Medicare patients), most Medicare Advantage plans operate on the concept of **managed care**. Different plans employ managed care principles to different extents and in different ways. In principle managed care means you have a primary care doctor (your PCP—an internist or family physician) who coordinates all your care. You see her for preventive health visits and when you're sick. She orders laboratory studies when needed and makes referrals to specialists. However, even your PCP cannot order any test she wants or prescribe any procedures she wants—some must be preapproved by the plan's medical director or representative.

The term *managed care* has been a lightning rod ever since this approach to medicine arose in the private sector, so let's get right to the pros and cons of the Medicare version. The following points will help you determine whether managed care in general may be right for you but also what to look for in a specific Medicare Advantage plan.

FINANCIAL CONSIDERATIONS

There are obvious cost savings under managed care. Since your primary care doctor may be able to handle many of your medical problems, some visits to specialists may be unnecessary. Managed care plans generally have panels of specialists who agree to provide care at specified fees. The same holds true for laboratories, hospitals, and other providers. MA plans that use managed care do reduce overall costs and are thereby able to pass along savings to plan members. In fact, certain types of MA plans can provide very reasonably priced solutions for their plan participants.

If you are on a fixed income where cost is the principal issue, an MA plan can offer comprehensive coverage at quite low expense. Given the costs of Medigap policies, there is almost no way that Original Medicare can be as inexpensive. Without a Medigap policy, the copay and coinsurance costs inherent in Original Medicare can add up rapidly; with a Medigap policy, the premiums for that policy must be factored in.

If you spend several months a year out of the country, Medicare Advantage may be a good choice for you because many MA plans include $50,000 foreign emergency coverage. Remember, Original Medicare has essentially no benefits for foreign medical care. You would need a Medigap plan that includes the foreign travel emergency benefit.

Then there are the pluses created by a competitive marketplace. Intense competition has given rise to a wide variety of features being offered that are not covered under Original Medicare. Prominent among these additional benefits are dental coverage and vision care. Some plans offer hearing aids at substantially reduced prices, a perk that many participants find extremely attractive. Gym memberships may also be included.

HEALTH BENEFITS OF COORDINATED CARE

But the cost-saving aspects of Medicare Advantage plans are not the whole story. Advocates of managed care believe that coordinated care is really superior care. They contend that requiring each enrollee to have a primary care physician who knows him well will lead to better outcomes and fewer errors. That doctor will not only be familiar with all of a person's medical issues and medications, but will also better understand him as an individual. Since all referrals to specialists originate with the PCP, results will funnel back to her and recommendations will be integrated more expeditiously into the patient's overall health plan. Dangerous drug interactions may be avoided more easily if one doctor controls all of a patient's medications. Of course, for this system to work maximally there must be trust and respect between patient and primary care physician.

AND THE TRADE-OFFS

What about the downsides? You must be comfortable with the restrictions placed on your choices by the specific MA plan. There should be relatively little disruption of your continuity of care under managed care if you're happy with your present PCP and she participates with the plan. But you should check to see if other doctors you see on a regular basis are in-network before opting for a particular Part C offering. Also, be very sure that your local hospital or a hospital that you would prefer to use if you're sick accepts the plan. Just because your PCP is on the staff of a particular hospital does not necessarily mean that the hospital is in the MA plan's network. If you need surgery, your surgeon might participate with the plan while the hospital or the anesthesiologist does not. Only after the surgery do you find out that your plan will not cover some potentially large bills.

Look first at which doctors and hospitals are in the networks of various MA plans available to you, but don't stop there. What about skilled nursing facilities if you need rehabilitation services after a hospitalization? Is there only one such facility on the panel? How far is it from your home? If you find that the plans you can choose from are too restrictive, managed care is probably not for you.

LOCATION

As opposed to Original Medicare, Medicare Advantage plans are often very location specific. Be careful if you live on the border of another state and sometimes get out-of-state medical care. A particular plan may have an extensive network of available providers where you live, but none at all across the state line. If this is your situation, look for plans with good out-of-network benefits, even if they cost more—or stay with Original Medicare. The same holds true if you travel to a major regional medical center for treatment of an unusual or complex medical condition. Specialized testing or therapies can be very expensive. Make sure you select a plan that assures you that your out-of-network coverage will specifically include services at that center. Otherwise, any savings you realized from joining the MA plan could disappear quickly.

⚠ **For those of you who live in two different parts of the country in different seasons, be especially careful!**

Snow-birds, this means you. If you're in Chicago for six months and Sarasota for the other six, an HMO plan with no out-of-network benefits would probably not be a good choice. For six months of the year you would have no coverage at all, except for emergencies. Be aware that many MA plans have very strict definitions of the term *emergency*. In some cases, you might have to contact the plan before receiving certain types of emergency care outside the plan's network.

For true, obvious emergencies, you will definitely be covered wherever you receive the emergency care, but you might have to return home for continued treatment. Let's say, for example, that someone who is 1,000 miles from home has a heart attack and is admitted to a coronary care unit. He does well but needs cardiac rehabilitation services after his discharge. The plan must pay for the hospitalization but easily could require that he return home for his rehab. This could even pertain in plans that have some out-of-network benefits, depending how broad or restrictive these benefits really are.

PROVIDERS IN FLUX

 The make-up of a plan's provider network can change rapidly.

Problems can arise when you select a particular plan because your PCP is included among its providers, only to find that he later chooses to cease participating or the plan cancels his contract. An example:

> In early October 2013, one of the nation's largest insurance carriers sent letters to thousands of physicians in at least 11 states notifying them that their contracts with the company's Medicare Advantage plans were being terminated as of February 1, 2014. The reasons were ambiguous but appeared to be cost-related. Patients were informed by letter that their doctors were being eliminated from the provider panels, but what were these patients to do? They could try to find new PCPs. If they wanted to keep their old ones, they could change MA plans, but the period during which they could transfer (the Open Enrollment Period) was October 15th to December 7th— not a lot of time. They could return to Original Medicare, but they'd have to find a Medigap plan during the same period— and they might be subject to medical underwriting. The result was confusion and dismay. All of this was possibly legal, but would you have wanted to be a patient in this situation?

Similarly, your PCP (or some other physician you see frequently) could elect to leave the plan, and you'd be faced with the same kinds of choices.

Deciding whether to choose Original Medicare or Medicare Advantage and, if the latter, which plan is clearly complicated, but the rest of this chapter will give you some information that I hope will help.

Your Costs in Medicare Advantage Programs

As mentioned earlier, if you join a Medicare Advantage plan, CMS will pay that plan a fixed monthly amount to cover your health benefits. But that doesn't mean you have no costs. Here's how it works:

Individuals who select MA plans, even though the plans are run by private insurance companies, are still responsible for Medicare Part A and Part B premiums. As you know, most people pay no premiums for Part A, but almost everyone pays the basic $104.90 monthly Part B premium; those with higher MAGI pay more. You pay these premiums directly to CMS whether you have Original Medicare or a Medicare Advantage plan. Similarly, income-related Part D extra premiums are payable to CMS whether a person has a free-standing Part D plan or drug coverage within an MA plan. Monthly premiums charged by the MA plan, if any, are in addition to the monthly payments to CMS. This is a common point of confusion.

⚠ **You must pay monthly Medicare premiums to CMS whether you participate in Original Medicare or an MA plan.**

In addition, there are costs related directly to your being a Medicare Advantage participant, including amounts you pay to the plan and cost sharing payments to providers. The plan may charge a monthly premium. There may be an annual deductible. There will almost certainly be copays and/or coinsurance for visits to doctors, laboratories, and hospitals. MA plans use these various cost sharing elements in all kinds of different amounts and combinations. Some may charge no monthly premium; some may have very different copays for primary care doctors versus specialists; some may have no copays for providers in their networks but significant ones for out-of-network care. The possible combinations are endless. Each plan also has an annual **Out-of-Pocket Spending Limit,** which is the absolute maximum you can pay in any given year, including all coinsurance, copays, premiums, and deductibles. After that limit is reached, the plan sponsor pays all bills. When considering joining an MA plan, you'll have to analyze very carefully which array of costs and benefits works best for you. Later on, we'll look more closely at how typical plans structure their payments. But before doing that, you need to understand the different types of available plans.

Types of Medicare Advantage Plans

Unlike Original Medicare, which is basically one program for everyone, MA plans can take many forms. These are distinguished largely by the extent to which they require coordinated care and how much flexibility you have in choosing providers.

Not only do plans differ from company to company, but numerous plan choices are frequently offered by individual insurance carriers. They will vary by premium costs, the manner in which cost sharing is structured, the amount of choice in selecting physicians, the degree to which coordinated care is required, how drug coverage is handled, and numerous other factors.

One major characteristic of Medicare Advantage programs of all types is their reliance on **provider networks**. Original Medicare allows you to see any provider who accepts Medicare's fee structure, and all providers in a geographic area are paid the same amount for the same service. Medicare Advantage plans function differently. Each insurance company that sponsors an MA plan creates a group of doctors, hospitals, skilled nursing facilities, laboratories, and other types of health care providers. Fees paid to these various providers are the result of negotiations and will often not be the same as Original Medicare's fees. Additionally, since each provider has a separate negotiated contract with a given plan sponsor, different doctors or hospitals may not necessarily be paid the same amount by a given plan. Sometimes there are financial incentives to physicians or groups of physicians for reaching certain quality-of-care measures or for keeping overall costs low. The resulting collection of health care providers who have contracts with a given plan sponsor is called its **provider network** or **provider panel**. Those who participate with a given plan are said to be **in-network**; those who don't are **out-of-network**.

There are six basic types of Medicare Advantage plans:

1. **Health Maintenance Organizations (HMOs)**—An HMO plan embodies the essence of managed care. You have a primary care doctor who coordinates your care. Referrals are required to see specialists. Each of your doctors, whether a PCP or specialist, must be a member of the HMO's provider panel. Similarly, hospitals, skilled nursing facilities, surgical centers, laboratories, and the like must be in-network. If you seek care outside the network or without a referral from your primary

care doctor, you may not be covered (except in emergencies). HMO plans are usually the least expensive. They provide comprehensive coverage at very low cost. There may be no monthly premium (aside from the premiums charged by CMS), and copays are generally quite low. Office copays for seeing a primary care doctor may be only $10–15, with preventive care visits often having no copay at all.

2. **Point of Service (POS) Plans**—POS plans are a variant of HMOs in which you have some coverage for going to doctors or hospitals outside the plan's network. You have a primary care physician who coordinates your care, and most of your providers should be in-network. You pay larger copays or coinsurance for going out-of-network. In-network referrals may or may not be required.

3. **Preferred Provider Organization (PPO) Plans**—PPOs provide one more level of choice in picking your providers. Generally you'll probably still have a primary care doctor, but referrals will not be required for you to see a specialist. You'll be able to go in-network or out-of-network, but you are encouraged to see the preferred providers; cost sharing will definitely be higher out-of-network. If POS plans and PPO plans sound somewhat similar to you, you're correct. There's a lot of overlap. What one company calls a PPO may resemble another's POS plan.

4. **Special Needs Plans (SNP)** —Unlike the first three plan types, Special Needs Plans are not available to everyone. Each SNP is designed to serve only a specific type of patient. Often these individuals require considerable amounts of care. They may be residents of nursing homes or other long-term care facilities, or they may have certain specific chronic diseases. Some qualify for both Medicare and Medicaid. The plans that provide this type of care are geared specifically for the particular patient population they serve. They rely heavily on coordinated care.

5. **Private Fee-for-Service (PFFS) Plans**—This relatively new option does not really utilize the principle of managed care at all, since there is no coordination of care. Most plans have no provider network. You are responsible for asking each doctor you see whether he is willing to accept the fees paid by your Private Fee-for-Service plan. If not, he may choose not to treat you (except in emergencies) or you may be responsible for his

entire bill. The same applies to hospitals and other providers. Some PFFS plans do have provider networks in which everyone has agreed to accept the plan's fees.

6. **Medical Savings Account (MSA) Plans**—This type of plan combines a high-deductible insurance policy with a special savings account set up at a bank. The plan deposits a specified amount of money (which is less than the deductible) into the bank account. You pay for medical services, including Medicare-covered services and also some services not typically covered under Original Medicare, from this account. Once you have spent the amount of the insurance policy deductible on Medicare-covered costs, the plan pays 100% of additional costs. This concept may sound familiar to many of you. It is analogous to the high-deductible plus HSA accounts often provided as employer-sponsored insurance.

Drug Coverage Under Medicare Advantage

In looking at various MA plans, you may find some that include drug coverage and some that don't. In recent years it has become more and more common for MA plans to include Part D–like drug coverage. Clearly, if you're looking for "one-stop shopping," it makes sense for medications to be part of the package. If a plan includes drug coverage, you will not have a separate Medicare Part D plan. The same rules that apply to Part D plans also pertain to drug coverage incorporated into MA plans, including the coverage gap. If you come upon a Medicare Advantage plan that you really like but that doesn't include medications, that's okay. You'll simply purchase a separate Part D plan. If drug coverage is not part of your MA plan and you don't buy a Part D plan, you'll be subject to the same penalties discussed in the preceding chapter.

MEDICARE ADVANTAGE AND MEDIGAP

Medicare Advantage plans are not designed to work with Medigap policies. As you will recall, Medigap policies are specifically designed to fill in the cost sharing gaps in Original Medicare. Since MA plans can take such a wide variety of forms, the rigid structure of Medigap policies simply won't work with them. In fact, it is illegal to sell you a Medigap policy if you're enrolled in an MA plan.

There is one situation in which you can have both an MA plan and a Medigap policy. If you've been on Original Medicare and decide to try an MA plan to see if you like it, you might consider keeping your Medigap policy and continuing to pay the premiums. You won't be able to use it with your MA plan, but you also won't be subject to medical underwriting if you decide to go back to Original Medicare. In this situation, you'll be wasting money paying for a policy you can't use (and Medigap policies can be expensive), but you'll be protecting yourself from the possibility of not being able to buy a Medigap policy once you've dropped it. Under guaranteed issue rights (discussed in Chapter 4), if you drop Original Medicare plus Medigap to try an MA plan, you can change back to Original Medicare and re-enroll in your Medigap plan, as long as you were in the MA plan for less than one year. For longer periods, guaranteed issue rights do not apply.

What Do Typical Medicare Advantage Plans Look Like?

How MA plans really work will become clearer with the help of some specific examples. The most commonly chosen plans tend to be HMOs and HMO variants. Let's look at two typical plans, one a pure HMO with no out-of-network benefits and the other a similar HMO with an added POS option. They're shown in the following table.

	PURE HMO	HMO WITH POS OPTION	
Plan's monthly premium	$ 0	$175	
Annual deductible	$ 0	$ 0	

COPAYS		IN-NETWORK	OUT-OF-NETWORK
Primary Care Office Visit	$15	$15	$40
Specialist Office Visit	$30	$25	$40
Routine Physical	$ 0	$ 0	$ 0
Preventive Services	$ 0	$ 0	$ 0
Labs, X-rays, other tests	$ 0	$ 0	20 %
Routine Vision/ Hearing Exams	$30	$25	$40
Outpatient Surgery	$175	$125	20%
Ambulance	$175	$175	$175
Urgent Care	$30	$30	$45
Emergency Room Care ($50,000 limit outside of U.S.)	$65	$65	$90
Inpatient hospital	$250/day For days 1–7 $0 for days 8+	$200/day For days 1–7 $0 for days 8+	$300/day For days 1--7 $0 for days 8+
Out-of-Pocket limit	$5,600	$5,600	$5,600

DRUGS

Deductible $150 (generic exempt)

	1 month	3 months	1 month	3 months
Tier 1: Generic	$10	$20	$10	$20
Tier 2: Preferred Brands	$40	$80	$40	$80
Tier 3: Non-Pref. Brands	$80	$160	$80	$160
Tier 4: Specialty Drugs	25% coinsurance		25% coinsurance	

In examining these premiums, copays, and coinsurance values carefully, several things become clear. For a basically healthy person, the costs involved in participating in the HMO can be extremely low. The plan charges no monthly premium. There is no annual deductible for medical care and only a $150 deductible for medications (but no deductible if all drugs are generic). Routine physical exams (which can be full physical examinations, unlike the "Wellness" exams of Original Medicare), laboratory tests, and preventive care are free. Copays for a few office visits to a primary care physician will not add up very quickly when copays are only $15. Two visits to specialists would add $60. Taking three generic medications will cost $240 per year. If outpatient surgery is needed, there's a $175 copay; that's all. The vision and hearing benefits are nice additions not included under Original Medicare, and the availability of $50,000 in emergency overseas coverage is reassuring for anyone who travels abroad. Even if major medical problems arise, the maximum personal outlay is $5,600. The biggest trade-offs versus Original Medicare are that all providers must be in-network, referrals to specialists are required, and many diagnostic tests and procedures must be preapproved by the plan.

For $175 per month ($2,100 per year) the option to utilize providers outside of the network can be added. Copays and coinsurance will sometimes be higher when going out-of-network. For many people, the ability to select doctors and hospitals from a much wider pool of choices is important. But the out-of-pocket maximum is still just $5,600. For them, the POS option may be worth the additional cost.

Comparing Plans

Unfortunately, it is extremely difficult to compare Medicare Advantage plans. The six plan types described earlier are disparate in concept and details. In addition, the various offerings available within any plan type will differ markedly. As noted, each plan will have its own premiums, deductibles, copays, and coinsurance. But they will also vary in their requirement for coordinated care, use of provider networks, and the makeup of those networks. Insurance companies may offer a plan in one geographic area but not in another.

The Medicare website can be of limited help. The same comparison tool discussed for evaluating Medicare Part D drug plans can be used to evaluate Medicare Advantage plans. Start by going to www.medicare. gov and follow the same steps used for Part D (outlined in detail in Appendix B). That is, click **Compare Drug and Health Plans** and go through all the steps regarding your medications and pharmacies. When you get to the page entitled **Step 4 of 4: Refine Your Plan Results**, go to the box on the right side and click the second and third choices (**Medicare Health Plans with drug coverage** and **Medicare Health Plans without drug coverage**). Then click on **Continue to Plan Results**.

You will now get to results that look strikingly like the ones you obtained when you went through this exercise for Part D plans. Much of the information will be about each plan's drug coverage and, unfortunately, very little about the medical coverage. In the fourth column, entitled *Health Benefits*, there is some rudimentary information about doctor choice and a figure for the plan's Out-of-Pocket spending limit. In the sixth column, entitled *Estimated Annual Health and Drug Costs*, there is a dollar amount. But what does it mean? The program knows your medications, since you've entered each of them. But how does it know anything about your overall health, how many doctors you will see, what laboratory tests you might need, or whether you'll be hospitalized? Not very useful.

Of much more interest is the seventh column, entitled *Overall Plan Rating*, where you'll find the star ratings. These are extremely important—much more important than the star rating for Part D plans. A Medicare Advantage plan will control your *entire health coverage*. How CMS and the plan's previous participants have evaluated a given plan may be your only objective measure in comparing different options. Beyond the data on star ratings, there isn't a lot in these tables to help you with your choice. Sadly, the **Medicare Plan Finder** software is far less helpful in comparing Medicare Advantage plans than Part D plans.

The Preapproval Nemesis

There is one more issue that I've alluded to but not discussed, and it may be important in your decision-making process. Unfortunately, it's not something that you'll be able to research easily by reading plan brochures, websites, or documents. This has to do with restrictions on care. Most managed care plans require preapproval of certain specific tests, diagnostic procedures, operations, and other therapeutic interventions. Physicians must submit preapproval requests, and they can be denied by the plan. Many physicians complain that getting approvals for certain of these diagnostic and treatment options can be cumbersome, arbitrary, and frustrating. An MA plan is under no obligation to approve payment for any specific procedure. Indeed, the plan (usually through its medical director) can simply rule that a scan or operation is not medically necessary and deny it. Although there are appeals processes for requests that are denied, these can be time consuming and by no means always successful. An oft-sited example of one such procedure is a nuclear stress test to evaluate someone with possible coronary heart disease. Another is Magnetic Resonance Imaging (MRI) to diagnose knee, shoulder, or back pain. And there are others. I know of many physicians who have dropped out of MA plan panels, not because they were unhappy with the fees they were receiving but solely due to continual aggravation over the preapproval process. Obviously, the extent to which this could be a problem for you will depend heavily on the policies of the particular Medicare Advantage plan you are considering. I know of no way to evaluate this problem by reading plan materials.

The star rating system (described earlier) contains patient satisfaction as one of its components, but it's only one among multiple factors that make up the final score. If enough plan participants are unhappy with decisions made by the plan, this could show up in the plan's star rating. Since physicians are the ones who have to deal with preapprovals, physicians (and especially the office staff members who have to work at obtaining the approvals) are the most knowledgeable about this issue. Asking your doctor or the office manager about personal experiences with different plans may prove very insightful.

Using an Insurance Agent

Just as you can use an insurance agent to help you purchase a Medigap Policy or Medicare Part D plan, you can seek such assistance in researching and enrolling in a Medicare Advantage program. A good agent can be a very useful resource, especially in comparing the many plans available from multiple insurance companies. However, using an agent to purchase a Medicare Advantage program is not exactly the same as using an agent to buy a Medigap or Medicare Part D policy. Here's why: In all three cases, the policy is being sold to you by an insurance company and the agent receives a commission from the company for selling you the policy. It's legal and totally proper. Insurance agents provide a valuable service and deserve to be paid. But consider the following difference. Most people who can afford a Medigap policy will buy one. The main issues for them are which type of policy they want (such as Plan A versus Plan F) and which company provides the best value. Remember, all Plan F policies by law provide exactly the same benefits as all others. For individuals who neglected to buy a Medigap policy during their Initial Enrollment Period, medical underwriting issues will also need to be considered. Regarding Medicare Part D plans, almost everyone will need to select one, both because they provide important medication benefits and because there are substantial penalties for not doing so. Here, again, the only real question is which plan to choose.

It's different when it comes to deciding between Original Medicare and Medicare Advantage. If you choose Original Medicare, the agent receives no commission. CMS does not provide for any payments to insurance agents for Medicare Parts A and B. On the other hand, an insurance agent receives a significant commission from the private insurance company for enrolling you in one of its Medicare Advantage plans. The implications are obvious.

⚠️ **An agent will want to show you the positive aspects of Medicare Advantage plans, but not many of the negative ones.**

I'm not trying to steer you away from using an agent. On the contrary, I believe agents provide a very important service. Every insurance agent who sells Medicare Advantage plans must be registered with the insurance companies that underwrite them and must comply with the educational requirements of those companies, which involve courses and exams. This is particularly important when dealing with Medicare Advantage, since the plans differ so greatly. Evaluating the features of various specific plans is not easy. An agent can provide useful comparisons in costs and benefits. The feedback she has gotten from previous clients can give her invaluable insights into the relative ease of dealing with various MA carriers. I believe that a reputable agent can truly be of tremendous help.

⚠️ **As I've mentioned in earlier sections, make sure you know with whom you are dealing. Get recommendations from friends and family who have had experiences with agents. As with any industry, there will always be unscrupulous individuals who will try to get you to sign up** for things that you don't really understand. If someone is extolling the virtues of one company's plans to the exclusion of all others, beware. You want the ability to compare the pros and cons of a variety of plans.

Key Points for Medicare Advantage

- Medicare Advantage (MA) plans (also called Medicare Part C or Medicare Health Plans) are an alternative to Original Medicare chosen by almost 30% of those eligible for Medicare. A single plan covers inpatient and outpatient services of all types; most include medications.

- Plans are run by private insurance companies under Medicare guidelines. They must cover the same services as Original Medicare, but they may do so in different ways.

- CMS pays the Medicare Advantage plan a monthly amount to cover all the enrollee's care.

- All seniors qualify; no pre-existing condition exclusions.

- Enroll during the Initial Enrollment Period; or switch from Original Medicare any year during the annual Open Enrollment Period, with coverage beginning January 1st.

- Monthly premiums, deductibles, copays, and coinsurance can be used in varying combinations.

- There are many types of Medicare Advantage programs, but most emphasize coordinated care by a primary care physician.

- Each plan establishes a provider panel (provider network) made up of physicians, laboratories, hospitals, nursing facilities, and other medical agencies.

- Plans may be strict HMOs in which all care must be in-network or may allow care outside the network, usually with higher premiums and cost sharing.

- Drug coverage within an MA plan is similar to a stand-alone Part D plan, including formularies, tiers, payment stages, and the donut hole.

- Some diagnostic and therapeutic procedures are subject to preauthorization by the plan. The preapproval process may be difficult, and requests may be denied; appeal processes are available.

- The make-up of a plan's provider panel can change rapidly. One or more physicians or other providers may leave the plan or be excluded by the plan, leaving patients without access to their regular doctors.

- Plans vary so greatly that comparisons can be difficult. Using an insurance agent who represents several companies may save you time and provide insights into the benefits and liabilities of the different options.

- Beware of hard sells by plan representatives; know with whom you are dealing.

Bottom-Line Recommendations:

- An HMO-type Medicare Advantage Plan provides the least expensive way to obtain comprehensive medical coverage for a Medicare recipient. Out-of-pocket costs can be extremely low under this option.

- For those desiring a greater choice of providers, compare the costs of Medicare Advantage POS and PPO plans with the cost of Original Medicare plus a Medigap policy. Take into account premiums and cost sharing. You will have to make some assumptions regarding how much medical care you may need.

Chapter 7

An Outline for Decision-Making

Now that you've learned about all the subtleties of Medicare and had a chance to think about your various options, it's time for decision-making. Perhaps you've already figured out exactly what you want to do. If so, you may not need the following outline.

The available choices will depend on your age and whether or not you're already enrolled in a Medicare plan. They'll be different if you're approaching your 65th birthday than if you're older, so I'll break things down in that way.

Individuals Approaching Age 65 (and Not Already on Medicare)

You can begin enrolling three months before your 65th birthday, so start thinking about your choices well before that important day. Medicare coverage commences on the first day of the month after you've signed up (and have reached 65), so if you wait until your birthday to enroll, you'll have to wait a month for coverage to begin.

I. **Decide whether you want to sign up for Medicare at all.**

A. Almost everyone should enroll in Medicare Part A.

a. Free for most of you.

b. A good deal (though admittedly costly) for those who must pay a premium; penalties apply for late enrolling.

B. The major exception involves individuals covered by an employer-sponsored high-deductible insurance plan with an associated Health Savings Account (HSA). Once you enroll in any part of Medicare, no further contributions can be made to an HSA.

II. Decide whether you want to sign up for Medicare Part B.

A. The Initial Enrollment Period is the seven-month period that starts three months before your 65th birthday, includes your birthday month, and continues for three more months.

B. Part B carries a monthly premium. About 95% of enrollees pay the base rate; higher-income individuals pay more based on MAGI.

C. Those who are covered by employer-sponsored creditable insurance plans based on current employment may bypass the Initial Enrollment Period without penalty. They are entitled to a Special Enrollment Period, which runs for eight months beginning the month after employment ends or the employer-sponsored insurance terminates.

    a. Both the employed person and spouse qualify for the Special Enrollment Period.

    b. Retiree medical insurance plans and COBRA are excluded.

D. Failure to enroll in Medicare Part B carries substantial penalties.

    a. For every full 12-month period that you don't enroll in Part B, your subsequent monthly premiums will increase by 10%.

    b. Penalties remain in effect forever.

E. Enrolling in Parts A and B does not mean you are necessarily signing up for Original Medicare as opposed to Medicare Advantage.

III. Decide whether you want Original Medicare or Medicare Advantage.

A. If you opt for a Medicare Advantage plan:

a. Consider whether you want a pure HMO, an HMO with a POS option, a PPO, or even a Private Fee-for-Service Plan.

b. Examine the offerings from several different insurance companies offering plans in your area. Check to see which providers are included in various plans, focusing on doctors you already use or want to use. The same goes for hospitals. Check pricing of various plans.

c. Make sure to include consideration of drug plans (Part D plans). Most MA plans include Part D benefits. You can and should purchase a separate Part D plan if your chosen MA plan doesn't include one.

d. An insurance agent can be very helpful in researching, evaluating, comparing, and recommending MA plans.

B. If you opt for Original Medicare:

a. Having signed up for Medicare, your Part A and Part B coverage should be in place.

b. Decide whether you want a Medigap policy.

(1) Your Medigap Open Enrollment Period is the six-month period that begins after you turn 65 and have enrolled in Medicare Part B.

(2) Determine how much coverage you want and which lettered plans interest you.

(3) Contact your state insurance office for information on what plans are available in your state and a list of companies selling plans in your area. They will also be listed at the back of your copy of the Medicare handbook *Medicare and You* and at www.Medicare.gov/find-a-plan.

(4) Remember that all Medigap plans of a particular letter provide exactly the same coverage. Price should be your major criterion in choosing a plan.

     (5) Consider a high-deductible Plan F—it will be the least expensive and possibly the best overall deal.

     (6) An insurance agent can be very helpful in researching costs and comparing options.

  c. Decide whether you need a Medicare Drug Plan—Medicare Part D.

     (1) The Open Enrollment Period is the same as for Part B.

     (2) You may elect not to enroll in Medicare Part D if you have creditable insurance that covers medications. The insurance can derive from current employment or a retiree plan (which is different from the rules for Part B).

     (3) If you fail to enroll in Medicare Part D, penalties of 1% per month for every month you delay signing up will be assessed when you finally do enroll. Penalties continue indefinitely.

     (4) Assemble a list of all your medications and use the *Medicare Plan Finder* online software to evaluate available drug plans in your area.

     (5) An insurance agent can be very helpful in researching and comparing plans, including assisting you with using the *Medicare Plan Finder*.

Individuals Past Age 65

For the purposes of the following discussion, we'll assume that you have enrolled in Medicare and have at least Medicare Part A, which almost everybody should have.

  I. If you've been covered by an employer-sponsored plan based on current employment, you are entitled to enroll in Medicare Part B during a Special Enrollment Period, which extends for eight months beyond the month that your employer-sponsored coverage ended. All your choices are identical to those of a person approaching age 65, as detailed above.

II. If you neglected to enroll in Medicare Part B and weren't covered by an employer-sponsored plan based on current employment, you may enroll in Medicare Part B during any General Enrollment Period, which runs from January 1st through March 31st of every year. Your Part B coverage will begin on the following July 1st.

    A. You will be assessed penalties for failure to enroll at the proper time. Your Part B premium will be increased by 10% for every 12-month period that you could have enrolled in Part B but didn't.

    B. You are entitled to purchase a Medigap Policy during a Medigap Open Enrollment Period, which begins when you enroll in Medicare Part B and runs for six months. You can purchase a Medigap policy under the same conditions as if you had purchased the policy at age 65.

    C. You can purchase a Medicare Part D drug plan. If you had creditable drug coverage, no penalty will be assessed. It doesn't matter whether the creditable coverage was provided by a work-related plan, a retiree plan, or any other source.

    D. You can choose to enroll in a Medicare Advantage plan if you desire.

III. If you are already covered by Original Medicare Parts A and B or by a Medicare Advantage plan, you have the right to change plans once a year (every year if you wish to).

    A. You can change during the period October 15th through December 7th; the new coverage becomes effective the following January 1st.

    B. You can change into a 5-star rated Medicare Advantage plan at any time during the year.

    C. If you have Original Medicare:

a. You can select any Medicare Advantage plan of your choosing.

b. You will no longer be able to use any Medigap plan you have purchased.

(1) If you remain in the Medicare Advantage plan for more than one year and elect to return to Original Medicare, you will not be entitled to purchase a Medigap policy without medical underwriting.

(2) To cover this possibility, you can continue to pay premiums on your Medigap policy while in the Medicare Advantage plan, but you can't use it.

c. Your Part D coverage will move to the Medicare Advantage plan if it includes drug coverage; if it doesn't, you can keep your previous Part D plan or select a new one.

D. If you have a Medicare Advantage plan:

a. You can switch to any other Medicare Advantage plan available in your area. No restrictions. If the old plan included drug coverage and the new plan doesn't, you can purchase a separate Medicare Part D plan.

b. You can switch to original Medicare Parts A & B.

(1) You may want a Medigap policy to augment your coverage.

a) If you have been covered by Medicare Advantage for more than one year (one plan or more than one), you are not entitled to a Medigap Open Enrollment Period and can be subject to medical underwriting.

b) If you have been covered by Medicare Advantage for less than one year, you have guaranteed issue rights and can choose any Medigap plan available in your area without medical underwriting.

    c) You may also have guaranteed issue rights for other reasons:

- Your MA plan withdrew from Medicare or stopped writing policies in your area.

- Your MA plan has failed to follow the rules or misled you.

(2) You will need a Medicare Part D drug plan.

    a) If your MA plan contained drug coverage, you can purchase a separate Part D plan to provide drug coverage.

    b) If you had a separate Part D plan while on MA, you can keep that plan or change to a new one.

    c) No penalties since the previous coverage would be deemed creditable.

IV. If you are covered by Original Medicare, you cannot normally obtain a Medigap plan beyond the Medigap Open Enrollment Period without being subjected to medical underwriting, possible exclusion of preexisting conditions, and even inability to get a policy at all. However, under certain circumstances, guaranteed issue rights apply and you can get a policy without conditions. These include:

A. You have been covered by an employer, union, or retiree insurance plan (including COBRA) that provides secondary coverage to Original Medicare, and that plan ceases to exist or you no longer qualify for it.

B. Your Medigap carrier goes bankrupt or you lose coverage through no fault of yours.

C. You move to a new area where your Medigap carrier doesn't write policies or the rules governing Medigap policies are different.

Testing Your Understanding

Now that you know all about Medicare, I'd like you to look at the following three vignettes. They're fictitious, but they illustrate the kinds of problems continually faced by Medicare enrollees. You'll find the answers on the following pages, but you probably won't need them.

1. Michelle and Fred Werner

Michelle and Fred, now both 68 years old and about to celebrate their 43rd wedding anniversary, had long and rewarding careers at the same aerospace company. Fred, an engineer, had decided not to retire at age 65. At that time, he'd been in the middle of an exciting project and enjoyed working with his team of gifted co-workers. The company was happy to keep him on—his ability as a leader was hard to replace. Michelle had been an accountant and had also liked her work, but she had lots of things she wanted to do in retirement and felt that age 65 was the right time for her. So, for the last three years Fred had remained on the company's medical insurance plan and Michelle was receiving benefits from the retiree medical plan, which was quite generous.

Both had delayed starting Social Security—they didn't need the money now and subsequent checks would be larger if they waited. But both had signed up for Medicare Part A when they turned 65. No reason not to. It cost them nothing and provided some additional insurance coverage.

Just about the time that Fred decided to retire, the company markedly scaled back the retiree medical plan. It was simply becoming much too expensive to maintain. Now it would <u>supplement</u> Medicare, not provide total coverage. No problem, they thought. They would both enroll in Medicare Part B as of July 1st. But when they contacted Social Security to sign up, they found that their two situations were very different. What had happened?

2. John Tompkins

John had been remarkably healthy all his life and had even run a marathon at age 61. About to turn 65, he was just signing up for Medicare. He'd been without medical insurance for 3½ years, ever since his employer had transferred operations overseas. But everything had been fine. He hadn't needed to see any doctors—just his glasses. His blood pressure was great.

He had already started receiving Social Security, so signing up for Medicare Parts A and B had been automatic. A friend told him he'd need to get a drug plan, which annoyed him, since he took no medications at all. He found one that was fairly cheap. OK. He was set.

About five months later, he started experiencing belly pains. He saw an internist and then a couple of subspecialists. John had a CT scan and a colonoscopy, both at the hospital, and some other tests he couldn't really remember. When he was ultimately diagnosed with colon cancer, he needed surgery and then month after month of chemotherapy—and that part wasn't over yet. The hospital and all his doctors accepted Medicare assignment. But when bills started arriving at his house, he stared at them in disbelief. They were huge. How could that be? He had Medicare. What was happening to him?

3. Anna Suarez

When Anna turned 65, she researched her options quite carefully and then joined an HMO-type Medicare Advantage plan from a national insurance company. It had a very large provider panel that included her family doctor and several specialists she had seen in the past. Anna was living on a fixed income and appreciated the plan's low cost. Preventive care visits, she noted, had no copay at all.

After 2½ years in the plan, she developed weakness and fatigue and was subsequently diagnosed with an autoimmune disease. Her family doctor referred her to an in-network rheumatologist, but she also wanted to see a specific physician at a large regional medical center, which was only 20 miles away but located in a different state. None of the doctors there were in her network. She had a consultation anyway and paid out-of-pocket. The visit and some associated tests were very expensive, but she really liked the doctor and wanted to get her care there.

It was August 10th, and she believed she could change plans once a year. She considered switching to Original Medicare and purchasing a Medigap policy, as well as moving to a different Medicare Advantage plan that allowed her to go out of network. What issues would she need to consider in making her choice?

Shown below are the answers to the questions raised by the three vignettes.

1. Michelle and Fred

Since Fred was receiving his medical insurance through his current employment (and it was creditable), he was entitled to a Special Enrollment Period when he retired. He could enroll in any Medicare program without penalty.

On the other hand, Michelle's insurance was provided by a retiree plan, so she was not entitled to a Special Enrollment Period. When she applied for Medicare Part B, she was assessed a penalty of 10% for each 12-month period that she hadn't been enrolled in Part B, starting at her 65th birthday. This came to 30% and would be assessed each year indefinitely. There was no Part D penalty, since her retiree insurance was creditable.

2. John

John had neglected to purchase a Medigap policy, so the bills he was receiving were for the cost sharing that was his responsibility. Although all his providers were participating and therefore accepted Medicare's fee schedule, copays and coinsurance can add up rapidly for expensive cancer therapy.

With a diagnosis of cancer, John would have difficulty buying a Medigap policy. He could choose to switch to a Medicare Advantage plan, which would take effect on the following January 1st, but he might have to change his doctors or the facilities where he was receiving treatment.

3. Anna

One option for Anna would be to switch to a Medicare Advantage plan that includes out-of-network benefits. Her premiums would be higher, but the plan would help pay for her care at the out-of-state medical center. Since MA plans are generally state specific, it's unlikely she could find one that includes that institution in its provider network.

She could change to Original Medicare, but she would have trouble finding a Medigap plan that would cover her autoimmune disease. Since she had been in an MA plan for more than a year, she does not have guaranteed issue rights.

How did you do? If you answered the questions accurately, you've got a good base of knowledge about your options and can use the following worksheet to record the course of action you intend to take, whether now or in the future. Should your circumstances change, you can always come back to this form and fill it out again. This worksheet is obviously an optional tool, useful only if you feel it will help you think through your decisions and/or have a place to refer to them at another time.

Decision-Making Worksheet

I AM APPROACHING AGE 65 AND...

☐ **My current insurance includes contributions to an HSA, so I cannot sign up for Medicare.**

☐ **I am not making contributions to an HSA but <u>do not</u> wish to sign up for Medicare at this time for these reasons:**

_____

_____

_____

Review the pros and cons of enrolling in Medicare to make sure this decision is correct for you. If it is, you're done for now. If your circumstances change, come back to this form and reconsider.

I AM APPROACHING AGE 65 AND WISH TO ENROLL IN MEDICARE.

☐ **I plan to sign up for Medicare Part A during my initial enrollment period.**

My initial enrollment period begins on   ____/____/____

My initial enrollment period ends on   ____/____/____

☐ **I plan to sign up for Medicare Part B . . .**

      ☐ during my initial enrollment period.

                    OR

      ☐ sometime in the future during a special enrollment period, which will run for eight months after I retire or my employer-sponsored insurance ends.

      ☐ I know when my current employer-sponsored insurance will end, so I must enroll in Part B by ____/____/____ to avoid paying a penalty.

☐ **I plan to select Original Medicare for my insurance coverage**

      ☐ I plan to purchase a Medigap policy.

My Medigap open enrollment period ends on (six months after I have signed up for Part B)   ____/____/____

Before my open enrollment period ends, I will identify the best Medigap plan and policy for me by . . .

❑   doing the research myself

❑   working with an insurance agent

❑   both

❑   I also plan to enroll in Medicare Part D.

My Part D Drug Plan open enrollment period ends on (the same date as for Part B)   ____/____/____

❑ **I plan to select a Medicare Advantage plan for my insurance coverage**

❑   I plan to choose an HMO.

❑   I plan to choose a PPO.

❑   I plan to choose a POS.

❑   I plan to choose a private fee-for-service plan.

I will identify the best MA plan for me by . . .

❑   doing the research myself

❑   working with an insurance agent

❑   both

❑   The MA plan I have decided to enroll in does not include drug coverage, so I plan to enroll in a separate Medicare Part D plan.

☐ **I AM OVER AGE 65 AND . . .**

☐ <u>**I HAVE NOT ENROLLED IN MEDICARE PART A.**</u>

I will need to enroll in Part A during the period ___/___/___
___/___/___

☐ <u>**I HAVE ALREADY ENROLLED IN MEDICARE PART A (OR AM NOW ENROLLING IN PART A) AND WISH TO ENROLL IN PART B.**</u>

> ☐ I was covered by an employer-sponsored plan and can enroll in Part B without penalty.

> OR

> ☐ I was <u>not</u> covered by an employer-sponsored plan and can now enroll during the general enrollment period of 1/1/201_ and 3/31/201_ but will have to pay a penalty of 10% for every 12-month period I was not enrolled.

> ☐ I plan to purchase a Medigap policy during the Medigap open enrollment period, which for me is the six months starting when I sign up for Part B.

> ☐ I plan to purchase a Medicare Part D plan. I may be subject to penalties if I did not have creditable drug coverage prior to signing up.

Part II

Using Your
Medicare Plan

Now That You've Got It, How Do You Use It?

OK. You've made decisions regarding your Medicare coverage and now you're a fully enrolled Medicare recipient. Whatever plan you've chosen, you're going to have to learn how to function effectively in that system. Each Medicare option has its own rules. You will need to fully understand them. Mistakes can be costly.

Do not assume that you understand how your Medicare insurance works just because you've had medical insurance in the past. No private insurance plan works the way Original Medicare does, and even Medicare Advantage plans, which are modeled after commercial managed care plans, will have differences since they must operate within Medicare-determined parameters.

In the remainder of this book I'm going to discuss how to maximize your medical care within the limits of what Original Medicare or your Medicare Advantage plan allows.

- What about your doctors? It's critical to have a primary care physician (PCP). Depending on the choices you've made, you may not be able to stay with some or all of your current doctors. How will you find new ones? Perhaps you've heard of Concierge Medicine—what's that all about?

- Hospitals can be scary and anxiety-provoking places. How do you choose a good one? Medicare has a unique approach to paying hospitals, which can significantly impact your hospital stay. What do you need to know about this?

- Skilled nursing facilities versus plain old nursing homes—what's the difference according to Medicare? Will any of it be covered? You need to know the rules, which are very specific. You also need to know about continuing care at home if you can't take care of yourself and possibly about how Medicare covers hospice care too.

- You'll need to keep good records and carefully check bills you receive from providers plus Explanation of Benefits forms from Medicare and other insurance carriers. You need to know how to appeal decisions made by insurance companies and medical facilities. And you'll have to watch out for Medicare fraud. I'll teach you how to do that too.

Some of these issues are unique to Medicare while others apply more broadly to the medical care system as a whole. In all cases, however, emphasis will always be on how the medical care system impacts care for seniors.

Chapter 8

Medicare, Your Doctors, and You

Willy Richardson was getting very frustrated. Twice in recent months he had been taken to the emergency room, and each time they had asked him who his regular doctor was. They told him he needed ongoing care to prevent these emergency visits, but he was having trouble finding a doctor. Friends had told him about several of their doctors. When he called them, though, some weren't accepting new patients at all, and others wouldn't see new Medicare patients. One doctor's receptionist even told him Medicare didn't pay enough to make it worth seeing Medicare patients. That didn't seem fair. He had always thought that Medicare would provide him with security for his "golden years," but his situation didn't seem golden at all.

Everyone needs a PCP!

PCP stands for **primary care physician.** As the name implies, this is the doctor you see <u>first</u>—for your annual exams, for preventive care, and when you're sick. Most PCPs who treat adults are either **internists** or **family practitioners**. Some have subspecialized in geriatrics, a field that emphasizes the unique problems and needs of aging patients. They're called **geriatricians**. See the following box for information on who may qualify to be your PCP.

Who Can Be My PCP?

Most PCPs are doctors, but more specifically they're physicians, since many types of medical professionals can be called doctors, including podiatrists, optometrists, clinical psychologists, and others. Physicians can have only two specific degrees: MD (Doctor of Medicine) and DO (Doctor of Osteopathic Medicine).

- **MD**—The vast majority of the doctors you will consider when choosing your PCP are MDs. Similarly, most medical and surgical specialists also have MD degrees. They attend college, then four years of medical school, and finally complete at least three years of postgraduate training called *residency*. When most people think of "doctors," they're thinking about MDs.

- **DO**—Known as *osteopathic physicians,* their training historically emphasized imbalances in the spine and muscles as causes of disease. In addition, holistic medicine—looking at the entire patient as opposed to specific diseases—was emphasized. Today the medical education of a DO is similar to that of an MD, with some continued study of spinal manipulation. Licensure requirements are also similar. Approximately 7% of physicians in the United States are DOs.

The vast majority of you will have either an MD or a DO as your PCP. But some nonphysicians can fill the role of a PCP. These include APRNs and PA-Cs:

- **APRN**—Nurse practitioners (Advanced Practice Registered Nurse) have taken advanced training and received either a master's or doctoral degree in nursing and have passed a national certifying exam. APRNs philosophically follow the nursing model, which emphasizes wellness and often attracts them to primary care. State laws determine whether an APRN must practice in collaboration with a physician or may practice independently, and these laws vary by state.

- **PA-C**—Physician Assistants (Physician Assistant-Certified) attend college, go on for advanced education that is essentially abbreviated medical school, and then must pass a national certifying exam. In most states a PA-C can examine and treat patients but must do so in association with a physician. (Warning: Don't confuse a Physician Assistant, a highly trained medical professional, with a Medical Assistant—the person who puts you in an exam room, takes your pulse and blood pressure, and tells you that the doctor will be in shortly.)

At the present time, the United States has an inadequate supply of physicians working in primary care, a situation that is expected to worsen as the Affordable Care Act results in more Americans having health insurance. APRNs and PA-Cs are capable of providing primary care, especially in the context of larger structured organizations such as clinics, medical groups, and staff-model HMOs, where consultation with a physician is readily available. In fact, some of the newer models of medical care delivery rely heavily on APRNs and PA-Cs serving as PCPs.

You very well may already have a primary care physician. But some people believe they don't need one. They reason as follows:

"I don't need a family doctor. I have a lot of specialists, and whenever I need a doctor I call the appropriate one. Specialists know more about their own fields than PCPs do. I want to see the person who knows the most."

Bad idea! I have no difficulty with an individual having a list of specialists. I like specialists—I'm one. As a dermatologist, I appreciate that patients often know they have skin problems and want to come directly to me. That's fine. But as we age, it is important to have one doctor who knows us well and who oversees our care, which can become more and more complicated over time. A list of sensible reasons to have a PCP appears in the box below. If you're just enrolling in Medicare and don't have a PCP, now is a good time to develop a relationship with a physician or other provider who can serve this important role.

Why It's Wise to Have a PCP (Especially Once You're on Medicare)

- Calling a specialist directly assumes you know what's wrong with you. Is the pain in your arm coming from your shoulder joint or are you developing a blockage in an artery to your heart? If you call an orthopedist and wait a week for an appointment, what might happen to your heart while you're waiting? Or perhaps you call your cardiologist first because of some chest pain. What if it's really an ulcer?

What type of specialist will you call if all your muscles start aching? Do you have a serious disease, or is it a reaction to a cholesterol-lowering medication? You can waste a great deal of time going to the wrong specialist, no matter how expert he might be.

- Who will you call if you're simply feeling awful? Who's the specialist for that? Let's say it's 11:00 A.M. on Saturday. A specialist might have office hours; more likely you'll be told to call on Monday. Your PCP or an associate could easily be seeing patients; someone should at least be available to call you back. But if you're not an existing patient of a particular PCP or group, those doctors have no responsibility to see you or talk to you. You could go to the emergency room and wait six hours to find out you have a bad cold. You could use an immediate care center, but that's not a perfect replacement for a PCP.

- If you're discharged from the hospital and several of your medications were changed while you were there, you'll need someone to renew those prescriptions once you're home. If they are, for example, heart medications, and the only specialists you've been seeing are an ophthalmologist and a dermatologist, who's going to handle this?

- Last, but certainly not least, who will provide preventive care? Once you have Medicare, you're entitled to a free Welcome to Medicare Exam and annual Wellness Exams. Who will do those exams and provide you with needed immunizations? Who will talk to you about your weight, your eating habits, or smoking? Who will look at the big picture? The answers are all the same—your PCP.

Immediate Care Centers as PCPs under Medicare

What about using an immediate care center, sometimes called an **urgent care center**, as your PCP? In recent years, such centers have proliferated across the country. Usually located in storefront offices, they may be open 24 hours a day or at least have extended hours. They serve an important function by providing a convenient place to see a doctor for acute illnesses and minor emergencies, without having to deal with the lengthy waits and high costs of an emergency room. Original Medicare covers visits to such centers under Part B. Coverage by a Medicare Advantage plan will depend on the plan's rules and whether or not the center is in-network.

Some people choose to let such facilities function as their PCPs. This may not be a good idea for two reasons:

1. A PCP should be *one* person who knows you well. He works with you in treating your various medical problems and gets to understand how your body reacts to infections, stressful situations, and medications. Immediate care centers are often staffed by several doctors.

2. An important part of primary care is preventive medicine. Will the physician at the immediate care center be attuned to providing the examinations, immunizations, screening tests, and counseling that are covered without cost to you by Medicare?

However, if a single physician at an immediate care center is willing to be your PCP, including preventive care, then that arrangement could work for you. If the physician is Medicare participating, then Original Medicare will treat your primary care visits exactly the same as visits to a PCP in a more "traditional" office setting.

PCPs Under Medicare Advantage

If you have elected to join an HMO-type Medicare Advantage plan, then you already have a PCP or will be getting one soon. As discussed in Chapter 6, coordinated care is the cornerstone of their philosophy, and it's your PCP who provides it. In most such plans it's mandatory. Even if your MA plan doesn't absolutely require a PCP, you'll be encouraged to have one. In Original Medicare you don't have to designate a PCP. But whether you've selected MA or Original Medicare, you should have one. I do.

Primary Care via Concierge Medicine

Another option you have for a PCP is what is known as **concierge medicine.** This approach to getting a coordinator of your health care is not for everyone, because it is not covered by Medicare. So exactly what is concierge medicine? In its basic form, it's primary care medicine without insurance. Patients sign up with a doctor—usually an internist, but sometimes a family practitioner—who provides them with primary care and charges them a monthly or quarterly fee.

⚠ **Because the concierge physician is unlikely to be part of any provider panels, concierge medicine is incompatible with most Medicare Advantage plans.**

> *One day identical letters arrived for Julie and Doug Wilson. They were from Dr. Benson, their family physician for 18 years. He was changing the way he practiced and would no longer be accepting insurance of any type. Instead, he would provide all their general medical care for a fixed annual fee. He would spend as much time as each person needed, offer same-day appointments, and provide 24-hour access to him via his cell phone.*
>
> *Julie and Doug talked it over. "I like this idea," she said. "With my arthritis and diabetes, I could really use the extra time and attention. All my medical problems mean we can't travel anymore. I'd like to use the money we don't spend on travel to sign up."*
>
> *"OK, but not me, replied Doug. "I don't see doctors that much. My health is fine using my Medicare. I like Dr. Benson, but I suppose I'll need to find a new doctor."*

Concierge medicine is definitely controversial. Patients in concierge practices feel it's a return to truly personal medicine. Opponents call it elitist—which may be why it's sometimes called **boutique medicine**— and a drain on physicians available to treat all the people.

> IN MOST TYPES OF CONCIERGE MEDICINE, THE PHYSICIAN OPTS OUT OF ALL INSURANCE PLANS, MEDICARE INCLUDED, AND NO INSURANCE CLAIMS ARE FILED.

Concierge medicine was born when doctors began to feel that they were working for insurance companies, not their patients. With insurance paying the bills, they were unable to give their patients the time required for quality care; the insurance companies dictated what services could be provided and how much they would pay for each. Opting for a concierge practice allowed a physician to minimize paperwork and spend the time needed by each patient, while at the same time increasing his compensation.

Some patients loved the idea, because concierge medicine seemed to offer them more personal care—perhaps the type that harked back to an earlier era. Several varieties have become available, making this PCP option more appealing to individuals of varying needs and means:

1. In the prototypical concierge practices, a physician has 250–300 patients (versus about 2,000 in most primary care practices). Each patient is charged $2,500–$5,000 per year, depending to some extent on the geographic location of the practice. For this fee, the patient receives:

   - An annual complete physical exam

   - As many office visits as needed

   - Same-day and after-hours appointments

   - House calls

   - Access to the physician by cell phone 24 hours per day, 7 days per week

   - Some basic laboratory tests performed in-office

   Although this represents a typical arrangement, some variations occur. For example, two concierge physicians can team together—each having his own patients but splitting some of the cell phone coverage.

2. A second model involves a physician having a very small number of patients—perhaps 30 or 40—and charging a great deal of money, in the range of $20,000 to $25,000 per year. He accompanies his patients to diagnostic procedures and to

specialists' offices. He may be asked to fly across the country to see a patient. Very few people can elect this kind of concierge care.

3. The third model is the virtual opposite of the second. Fees are low, perhaps only $50 per month, which provides for office visits when needed, but omits some of the amenities. Questions may be handled by email. It's designed for the average person. Some individuals who join this type of practice have no medical insurance but need a family doctor for a reasonable price. Others have insurance but feel the modest extra cost of this type of concierge medicine is worth it. Some people who work unusual hours and need appointments at specific times find this arrangement indispensable. Clearly practices of this type must be far larger than those in the more typical model.

4. An additional model functions differently in that the physicians continue to accept insurance. They charge a concierge fee for extra services such as longer appointments, extended office hours, complete physical exams for Medicare patients, and 24-hour cell phone access. These physicians continue to bill insurance companies (including Medicare and Medigap) for office visits and related services. As a result, their concierge fees tend to be lower than those of the prototype concierge practice. Since these physicians have not opted out of Medicare, they have the option of seeing both concierge and nonconcierge patients. A hybrid practice of this type allows them to continue to care for some longstanding patients in addition to their concierge practice.

If you opt for any of these models of concierge medicine, you will still need Medicare Parts A and B to cover hospitals, emergency rooms, laboratories, surgery, and specialists. It would be foolish indeed to pay for concierge care and, at the same time, risk massive medical bills for surgery, extensive testing, etc. Original Medicare plus a Medigap plan provides this coverage. Again, however, Medicare Advantage and concierge medicine are not a good fit.

Clearly, choosing a concierge doctor is not for everyone. For most seniors, it's simply too expensive. Medicare cost sharing, whether paid out-of-pocket or through premiums for a Medigap plan, already places financial burdens on many seniors. How many can afford the even greater cost of concierge practice?

▶ *If you have minimal medical needs but need a PCP:* The low-cost third model above may work for you, especially if you need appointments at unusual times of day.

▶ *If you have more complex, time-intensive medical issues:* You, like Julie Wilson, might choose to spend your money getting the personal attention of a concierge doctor rather than on vacations that are no longer manageable or on other discretionary expenses.

The future of concierge practice is uncertain. Obviously, its success depends on sufficient patients having the desire and ability to pay for it. If its appeal lures too many doctors, some will not be successful in establishing a viable practice. My guess is that it will continue to thrive among certain groups and in certain areas of the country.

Finding a New Doctor

People who have moved frequently often note that one of the most difficult aspects of moving is finding new doctors and dentists (some include hairdressers!). The relationship between a doctor and a patient evolves over time. Ideally, the doctor learns about the nuances of the patient's medical conditions, about her personality, fears, and expectations; at the same time, the patient develops confidence that her physician is medically knowledgeable and understands her particular medical and emotional needs. How could this possibly be easily replaced? The answer, of course, is that it can't.

If you are picking a new doctor because you're not happy with the old one, the transition may be relatively easy. Since you didn't think much of your previous doctor, you will clearly be open to someone new. But if you're changing doctors because of moving to a new community, your doctor's retirement, or the dictates of a Medicare Advantage plan (or in the rarer case that your current PCP won't accept Medicare and so you have to move on), finding someone who lives up to your expectations can be challenging.

How do you go about it? It's definitely not easy. You're trying to find someone who is competent and compassionate and whose personal style meshes with yours. Ideally, his office is not far from where you live and transportation is good. Hopefully, he's taking on new Medicare patients. If so, does he accept Medicare assignment? Or is he on your Medicare Advantage plan's provider panel? Let's explore these issues.

COST CONSIDERATIONS

For many of you, one important factor in selecting your doctors will be financial. Put simply, it can cost you much more to see some physicians than to see others—depending on the coverage selections you have made and whether a given physician has chosen to accept assignment in Original Medicare or join a Medicare Advantage plan's provider panel. As we've discussed, Original Medicare places no restrictions on which doctors you may see. If a physician accepts Medicare assignment, you can go there and Medicare will pay 80% of the approved fee and you will pay the other 20% (or your Medigap plan will pay it for you).

If you've selected a doctor who doesn't accept Medicare assignment, you still have some coverage. His charges will be limited to 109.25% of Medicare approved fees. Medicare will pay 95% of each approved fee and you will be responsible for the difference. For those of you who have chosen a Medigap Plan F or G, the additional amounts will be reimbursed by your plan. But if you don't have any Medigap coverage or you have a Medigap plan other than F or G, your out-of-pocket costs can be considerable. Remember, only Medigap Plans F and G provide any coverage for services from nonparticipating providers.

⚠ **Be sure you understand how to calculate the costs of receiving services from providers who don't accept Medicare assignment—see Chapter 3.**

Of course, if your Medicare Part B coverage is supplemented by an employer-sponsored insurance plan or retiree benefit plan, the details of that policy will determine the extent of your coverage for participating and nonparticipating providers. Some of these policies are so-called **indemnity plans**, which simply reimburse you a fixed percentage of the amount Medicare doesn't pay. In such cases, you'll have coverage for all physicians, but since cost sharing is greater when seeing a nonparticipating one, you'll have to pay somewhat more out-of-pocket. Retiree benefit medical plans in particular can be structured in a variety of ways. Some may be high-deductible policies that don't pay anything until your out-of-pocket costs reach a certain threshold; then they pay 100%.

CAN I STILL GET ACCESS TO THE "BEST" DOCTORS?

Cost considerations aside, everyone would like to have access to doctors perceived as the best out there. What constitutes "best" for you will vary with your needs and preferences, but it's an unfortunate reality that selecting a PCP who accepts Medicare assignment may limit your choices and sometimes affect the quality of service you receive.

> *When Doug Wilson decided to find a new doctor rather than sign up for Dr. Benson's concierge service, he chose a doctor who was board-certified in internal medicine, had admitting privileges at Doug's preferred hospital, and was on a university faculty. Clearly he was up on the latest advances in internal medicine, and Doug thought he'd get good care. The first office visit went fine, although Doug felt a little rushed when he wanted to talk to the doctor about some new aches and pains. Dr. Watkins seemed to spend more time entering information into his electronic medical record (EMR) than really listening, and when he recommended a nuclear stress test, Doug couldn't help wondering whether it was necessary since he'd never had that test for the same problem before.*

You may come upon a doctor you feel would be a good fit for you, only to find that his practice is closed; he's simply not accepting any new patients. Unfortunately, this is most commonly the case for doctors who are perceived as "the best doctors." Additionally, you should be aware that some doctors, especially PCPs, specifically limit the number of Medicare patients they will accept. In recent years, a growing number of physicians have come to feel that Medicare's fees are inadequate and contend that they cannot make a living with a heavily Medicare practice. Only by mixing younger, privately insured patients with Medicare patients can their practices exist financially. As a result, they will either not see any new Medicare patients or restrict the number of such patients. Additionally, some even limit the number of new patients in pre-Medicare years (e.g., starting at age 55 or 60) they will take on, since these patients will soon be covered by Medicare. Most physicians continue to see their existing patients who become Medicare recipients. No matter what some cynics may contend, treating patients for many years and getting to know them well represents one of the true joys of medical practice, and most doctors are loath to stop serving a longtime patient.

HOW MEDICARE REMUNERATES DOCTORS DIRECTLY AFFECTS YOUR CARE

The way in which Medicare compensates doctors has a major impact on how an office visit is conducted. CMS determines a specific approved fee for every medical and surgical service. Medical visits, which make up most of a PCP's practice, are covered by what are known as Evaluation and Management codes (commonly called E & M codes). These codes take into account three main elements: (1) The amount of medical history taken by the physician, (2) the extent of his physical examination, and (3) the complexity of decision-making required. A combination of these three items determines how a particular office visit will be coded for submission to Medicare and therefore how much Medicare will pay. Documentation of everything that was done regarding all three components of the office encounter is mandatory and can be quite time consuming.

Medicare's rules regarding E & M codes are fundamental to understanding why physicians do what they do in the office. It's the reason they spend so much time entering quantities of marginally relevant information into their computers, as Doug Wilson experienced. For every E & M code, Medicare's rules stipulate how much medical history must be obtained and how many areas of the body must be examined, regardless of how relevant the information is to the particular problem. To be paid, the physician must document all of this required data. That takes time—time that could be better used actually talking with his patient.

Traditionally, Medicare's fees for diagnostic procedures and surgery have been substantially more generous than those for medical visits. PCPs perform few procedures and rely largely on E & M coded services for their compensation. Office visits for aging patients can be complex and lengthy, yet payments from Medicare may not be proportional to the time and effort expended. Not surprisingly, this has resulted in discontent among PCPs and contributed to their desire to see fewer Medicare patients.

HOW TO LOOK FOR A NEW DOCTOR

How you go about finding a PCP will depend in part on why you need a new doctor:

▶ *If your current doctor will not accept Medicare:* As noted above, this isn't that common, but it does happen. When it does, I believe that your physician has an obligation to help you find a new PCP. At the very least, he should supply you with a list of PCPs that he feels are good doctors and that he knows are accepting new Medicare patients. Preferably, he should use his knowledge of you and your unique medical issues to recommend someone who would be a particularly good fit for you. (Unfortunately, some doctors don't agree with my view.)

▶ *If you don't have a PCP:* The best method is to ask people you know. Some of your friends or coworkers certainly have PCPs. Ask who they like (and don't). When you have some names, call their offices and inquire about their policies regarding new Medicare patients and about accepting assignment.

▶ *If you're relocating upon retirement:* If you don't know the area well, and have no personal friends to ask for referrals, finding all the healthcare providers you might need can be a bit trickier. Lists of providers accepting new patients (and specifically new Medicare patients) can often be obtained from the local medical society, hospitals, and senior centers. If you're moving to a retirement community, they are likely to have information on local physicians who treat Medicare recipients. As you meet people, ask everyone about their PCPs. In this regard, medical personnel such as nurses (including retired ones) are particularly good sources. Some useful credentials to look for when evaluating a doctor include board certification and academic appointments at university medical centers, both of which speak to acceptance by the medical community of the doctor's expertise.

⚠ As obvious as it may seem, when you're choosing a new doctor, pay attention to ease of transportation, especially if you're relocating and don't know how easy it would be to get around without driving. (Perhaps you drive everywhere now, but what happens if your eyesight fails and you have to give up your car?) Plan for the future. It's a shame to have to leave an established and rewarding patient-doctor relationship because you simply can't get to the office anymore.

Choosing a Medicare Advantage Doctor

Most Medicare Advantage plans restrict your choice of physicians to some degree. This varies from plan to plan and is most characteristic of HMO-type plans. When you join an MA plan, you will have access to a list of the doctors who make up the provider panel—available in publications and on the plan's website. I suggest using the website, since provider lists can change rapidly and written materials easily become outdated. Unfortunately, sometimes even the websites (which theoretically can be updated continuously) are not totally current.

Requiring that you use only in-network providers may significantly restrict your available doctor choices. If you go outside the list of physicians in the network, coverage may be limited or nonexistent. In some plans (usually PPOs or POS plans), you are allowed to select doctors outside the provider panel, but there will often be greater copays or coinsurance. Check carefully with your plan. Ideally, you have done the proper research and selected your plan with full knowledge of which providers are and are not included and what rules you must follow.

It's unwise to select a PCP who is not a member of your provider panel. Medicare Advantage plans that emphasize coordinated care tend to structure their cost sharing such that it's much less expensive for you to see an in-network PCP. In many plans, PCP visits, especially for preventive care, have no copays at all. Additionally, in-network PCPs will be familiar with the specialists, laboratories, and hospitals that make up the provider panel and consequently will be better equipped to make the most appropriate in-network referrals when needed. If you are intent on choosing a particular PCP who is not part of an HMO-style MA plan's network, you would be well advised to select a different type of MA plan or opt for Original Medicare.

Physicians Who Reject Medicare

Some physicians have chosen to totally opt out of Medicare. These doctors not only won't accept Medicare assignment, they will not agree to be constrained by Medicare's limiting fees. Anyone who seeks treatment from one of these physicians must sign what's known as a **private contract**, acknowledging that she understands she will be responsible for the entire bill, that the amount charged can be whatever the doctor chooses to charge, and that Medicare will pay absolutely nothing toward these bills. Medigap plans, including F and G, will also pay nothing if a private contract is in effect.

Private contracts must be in writing and signed by both the physician and the patient (or legal representative). Federal law strictly regulates their content. Much of it relates to the patient acknowledging that none of the charges will be limited by Medicare's fee schedules, covered by Medicare, paid by any Medigap program, or subject to reimbursement in any way. Such agreements must state whether or not the proposed services can be obtained from other practitioners whose charges will be covered by Medicare. They must also indicate whether or not the doctor has been excluded from Medicare. Any physician who enters into a private contract with even a single Medicare patient cannot receive any payments from Medicare for any patients—that is, he cannot see certain patients under Medicare and others using private contracts.

⚠ **Signing a private contract is not the same as signing a form that indicates that a particular service might not be covered by Medicare.**

For procedures or tests that could be deemed "not medically necessary" according to Medicare's rules, a patient can agree to pay out-of-pocket, even though other services from the same doctor are covered by Medicare. Physicians who normally treat Medicare patients (whether they accept assignment or not) can provide and charge for "not medically necessary" services. This has no bearing on their status as Medicare providers. Patients receiving such services must sign a form called an **Advanced Beneficiary Notice of Non-Coverage (ABN)**, which pertains only to the specific procedure(s) and date(s) delineated on it. A copy of an ABN is shown on page 175 in Chapter 11, along with a more extensive discussion of what it means to sign that form.

Seeing Your PCP under Medicare

Once you're a Medicare recipient, an office visit with your PCP or a specialist won't be fundamentally different from what it was pre-Medicare. Symptoms, diseases, and treatments don't suddenly change when you turn 65. However, the dictates of a new insurance program (in this case, Original Medicare or an MA plan), can result in some changes, and you should be aware of them.

- When a doctor sends you for testing or to see a specialist, make sure you ask whether that provider accepts assignment under Original Medicare or participates in your Medicare Advantage plan. Doctors often have favorite labs or specialists who have always provided them with good service, but sometimes those providers won't accept your particular insurance program. If that's the case, request an alternative provider.

- You will most likely receive your medications under a Medicare Part D drug plan. Since so many different ones are available, and their formularies can vary so widely, your doctor may not know which drugs are covered by your plan and, if so, in which tiers they're located. If you are prescribed a drug that turns out to be much too expensive, ask your pharmacist why it was so costly and if there are alternatives. Perhaps your physician can prescribe an equally effective one that's in the formulary or in a lower tier. But you may have to ask. Providing your doctor with a list of similar drugs will make her work easier. Don't feel it's insulting to your doctor to do this—it's your money.

- CMS emphasizes the importance of electronic prescribing, since it decreases errors, and physicians are penalized for not doing so. As a result, today most Medicare prescriptions are transmitted electronically from the doctor's office directly to a pharmacy. You'll no longer get pieces of paper with undecipherable scribble to give to the pharmacist. Make sure your doctor knows precisely which pharmacy you want to use, including the specific location, since large chain pharmacies can have multiple branches in a city or town.

- No patient should ever ask her physician to do anything unethical or illegal. Who, you might ask, would ever ask a doctor to do something like that? The answer: People do it all the time! Remember, Medicare is a program run by the U.S. government and funded by federal tax dollars. A doctor's medical records are legal documents, as are the requests for payment that she submits to Medicare. Entering knowingly incorrect information into the medical record and submitting knowingly incorrect bills are fraudulent acts and violations of federal law. Penalties are substantial, including fines and even jail time for serious offenders.

  Yet some people blatantly ask their doctors to break the law. This happens most often when a physician explains that a service requested by a patient is not considered "medically necessary" by Medicare. "Doctor, can't you just write down a different diagnosis?" "Doctor, can't you say it was really necessary because I was having pain?" "Can't you say that the growth looked suspicious for cancer?" Another egregious example is asking a doctor to change the date of an office visit or procedure. "Doctor, my insurance just changed and I'm no longer covered for that kind of procedure; can't you backdate the charges so I'll get reimbursed?" Altering a date, simply, is fraud.

- In a similar way, asking your doctor to forgo your 20% coinsurance can also get him into legal trouble with Medicare. Here's why:

When your doctor agreed to see Medicare patients and be bound by Medicare's fees, he actually agreed that Medicare would pay him 80% of the Medicare-approved fee *or* 80% of his fee, whichever was less. Normally, the Medicare-approved fee is substantially less. However, if the doctor waives your 20% portion, he is actually lowering his total fee to 80% of the Medicare-approved fee. Medicare should technically pay him only 80% of the 80% he would normally get. Here's an example: Suppose Medicare's approved fee for a complex office visit is $200, so Medicare pays the physician $160 and you owe $40. If the doctor waives your $40, he is in fact accepting $160 as his total compensation. By his doing so, Medicare's responsibility actually drops to 80% of $160, or $128. He has received $32 too much from Medicare ($160 minus $128). Keeping the entire $160 is a violation of federal law. You might ask how CMS could ever know that he didn't collect your $40. In most cases, CMS never finds out. But if it does, and particularly if it ascertains that he has done this on a regular basis, he can be in substantial trouble. It could be considered Medicare fraud. As mentioned above, DON'T ask your doctor to do anything illegal.

Elective Surgery: Getting a Second Opinion

Joan Allen was anxious to see her friend Marilyn Regan. She was upset—very upset—and needed to talk. Just last week she had been diagnosed with cancer of her uterus—they had called it endometrial cancer—and was told she needed surgery. The diagnosis of cancer had shaken her badly. Earlier that day she had consulted the surgeon who'd been recommended by her PCP, but now she was even more apprehensive. The surgeon had explained what he felt needed to be done, but he hadn't said all that much and she had lots of questions—about her recovery, possible complications, the chance of being cured, and more. He hadn't answered them to her satisfaction.

"Marilyn, I know you went through the same thing two years ago. How did things work out for you?"

"I really liked my surgeon from the first time I met him. He was kind and compassionate—even had a sense of humor. The surgery went well and he was definitely there for me before and after it. His name is Dr. Rhee. I'll get you his number if you like."

"Absolutely. He sure sounds like the surgeon for me."

If you're contemplating elective surgery, it's never a bad idea to consider a second opinion—and, if the second opinion differs substantially from the first, even a third to help clarify why the initial two were so different. Seeking multiple opinions is fine when there appears to be disagreement among experts. What's not a good idea, however, is going from physician to physician until you find one who'll tell you what you've already decided you want to hear. Understanding how your Medicare plan, whether Original Medicare or Medicare Advantage, views second opinions is very important if you are contemplating surgery:

- Original Medicare definitely covers second surgical opinions. In addition, if the second opinion differs from the first one, Medicare will also cover a third opinion. All these surgical consultations are covered under Medicare Part B. You are responsible for the 20% coinsurance or for the higher coinsurance required if a surgeon doesn't accept assignment. A Medigap policy will provide additional coverage, depending on which lettered Medigap plan you have.

- If you have selected a Medicare Advantage plan, the exact rules regarding second surgical opinions will be determined by the plan. In general, MA plans cover second opinions and, in fact, encourage them. Some MA plans will actually require second opinions before they will approve certain surgical procedures and may require that the two opinions concur.

- Original Medicare does not presently restrict what surgical options you choose, as long as the procedure is medically necessary. MA plans, on the other hand, are not obliged to authorize surgery just because you want it or your physician recommends it. In this setting, second opinions may be instrumental in determining whether a plan allows or denies coverage for a particular procedure.

Chapter 9

Medicare, the Hospital, and You

Ernie Jones had been getting more frequent chest pain when he exercised. A stress test had shown heart artery blockages and the cardiologist had told him he needed cardiac bypass surgery. Heart surgery was now being done at his local hospital (for about a year); but Ernie wasn't sure that was for him. Wouldn't it be better to go to a larger medical center where that type of surgery had been done for many years? He knew that his Original Medicare coverage would allow him to choose either hospital. He would talk to his PCP and research his options — but he knew he had to do it quickly.

Medicare covers "medically necessary" use of a hospital, whether it is a trip to an emergency room or an admission for surgery. Both emergency and elective treatments are included. As is always true with Original Medicare, you have your choice of providers—in this case, any hospital that participates with Medicare. In Medicare Advantage programs, there may be restrictions on which facilities you can use for elective procedures. If you don't use an in-network hospital, you may have larger copays or deductibles, or in some cases you may not be covered at all.

⚠ **It is imperative to check with your Medicare Advantage plan prior to any nonemergency trip to a hospital. Don't rely on a brochure or even the plan's website. Make sure to get verification from the plan that the facility you will be entering is definitely in the plan's network.**

Emergency trips to the hospital are handled differently. CMS regulations require all Medicare Advantage plans to cover you in any hospital for emergency services. So if you're taken by ambulance to a hospital for, say, severe chest pain or an accident, you don't have to worry about your coverage.

How Medicare's System for Paying Hospitals Affects Your Inpatient Care

Earlier we talked about how Medicare's methodology for paying physicians has affected how office visits are conducted. It's equally useful to understand how hospitals are paid, since Medicare's payment system for inpatient services has a major effect on hospital care. Why does everyone seems to leave the hospital so quickly? Why are patients transferred so rapidly to convalescent homes to finish their recovery? Why can't you stay in the hospital an extra day if there's no one to pick you up? Wouldn't it be beneficial if you could remain hospitalized for a couple more days to regain your strength? The answers to all of these questions are the same:

> IF YOU ARE AN ORIGINAL MEDICARE PATIENT, THE HOSPITAL IS NOT PAID BY THE DAY; RATHER, IT'S PAID BY THE *REASON YOU'RE THERE.*

This may seem strange. In the chapter on Medicare Part A, we talked about how Medicare counts the days you're in the hospital. For the first 60 days, there are no copays. Beyond 60 days, daily copays apply; and beyond 90 days, copays increase and the "lifetime reserve" comes into play. All of this suggests that "days in the hospital" determines Medicare's payments to hospitals. Not so.

Prior to October 1982, Medicare paid a hospital according to that hospital's costs in caring for a patient. Each day in the hospital, each lab test, each operation, each medication, each bottle of IV fluid—all were billed to Medicare as separate items. A hospital simply submitted a detailed bill to Medicare and each service or item was paid for. But it became clear that this payment system was getting vastly too expensive, with no incentive for hospitals to become more efficient or control costs. So Medicare changed the way it pays hospitals. Since 1982, Medicare has employed what is known as a **prospective payment system.** Under this system, hospitals are not compensated for what is actually done but rather by what Medicare deems to be an appropriate global payment for each patient's particular medical problem and required treatment.

DRGS REIGN

You may hear the term **DRG** (Diagnosis-Related Group), which is the specific methodology employed. Every patient's hospital admission is assigned a payment category according to the admitting diagnosis and anticipated treatment, along with some additional factors that might complicate the hospital stay, including the patient's age, general health, and certain specific medical conditions. At present, there are about 1,000 DRG categories. The system is said to be *prospective* because the DRG is determined from information at the time of admission. Medicare pays the hospital only the amount dictated by the DRG (with some exceptions; see the box on pages 144-145). That's it. It doesn't matter whether the hospitalization lasts three days, five days, seven days, or two weeks. Let's look at an example:

> *Doris Winberg fell stepping off a curb. In the emergency room she was diagnosed with a broken hip and admitted to repair the fracture. The plan now is to operate and insert a metal hip bone replacement. Doris is 86 years old with diabetes and high blood pressure. She takes blood thinners because of a possible mild stroke a year ago. The DRG determination includes the diagnosis (fractured hip), the planned procedure, Doris's age, and the potentially complicating medical conditions and medications. If the operation goes smoothly and Doris does beautifully, she will be able to go home fairly quickly.*

> *But what happens if Doris develops a temperature of 102 degrees? Tests have to be done to determine whether she has an infection and, if so, where. Bacterial cultures must be taken and X-rays done. It's found that she has developed an infection at the surgical site, so she needs antibiotics and perhaps a local procedure. She ends up staying in the hospital for 10 days—far longer than initially planned. Medicare's DRG payment to the hospital is the same for both scenarios.*

MEDICARE'S EFFICIENCY MEASURES MAY ACTUALLY PROTECT YOU

If you end up hospitalized and are afraid the hospital will callously discharge you prematurely, trying to save money at the expense of your health, it may be reassuring to know that the emphasis on efficiency is not all bad.

1. These days, hospitals are working harder and harder at preventing complications, which significantly increase the length of hospital stays and necessitate costly tests, complex nursing care, additional procedures, and numerous other expenses for the hospital. Obviously, this is good for patients too. Reducing complications is a major win-win, keeping costs down for the hospital and keeping you healthier.

2. To prevent the need for readmissions created in some cases by shorter hospital stays, hospitals nationwide are also implementing programs to follow patients more closely post-discharge and to find new and creative ways to assure adherence to post-discharge medication regimens, proper diet, and therapy programs. One result of shorter hospital stays is that many patients have not totally recovered when they are discharged. Some end up having to be readmitted to the hospital for additional treatment, especially if they have not received adequate post-discharge continuing care. Until recently, such readmissions did not represent a financial problem for a hospital. If a patient had to return to the hospital, the new admission generated a new DRG payment from Medicare. There was no incentive to find ways to limit returning to the hospital. As of October 2012, however, CMS initiated a new program whereby hospitals are penalized for too many readmissions. Specifically, if a hospital is deemed to have an excessive readmission rate, it could be assessed a penalty of up to 1% of total payments on all Medicare patients for the next year. By 2015, this will rise to a maximum of 3%, which represents a lot of money for a hospital and serves as a strong incentive to control readmissions.

The programs that a hospital employs will often be diagnosis-specific. For example, a major disease for which readmissions is a problem is congestive heart failure. So a hospital may implement an aggressive follow-up program for this condition; but if you have a different diagnosis, this program's existence will be irrelevant to you.

⚠ **If you have a good primary care physician who is on top of your specific problems, she will provide follow-up. Ideally, the hospital will have informed her about your discharge in a timely manner. But discharges can be quick and mistakes happen, so I strongly recommend you also contact her office to let her know you're now out of the hospital.**

Exceptions to the DRG rules:

- Extremely lengthy hospitalizations caused by unusual events and extenuating circumstances are handled differently by Medicare.

- The DRG payment system applies only to "acute care hospitals," which are the typical community hospitals and medical centers that treat trauma, medical illnesses, problems requiring surgery, cancer treatments, etc. Specialized hospitals such as rehabilitation hospitals and psychiatric hospitals have their own rules.

- Very small hospitals, which are mostly in rural areas, are exempt from DRGs; they are paid in a more traditional manner based on their costs.

Hospital Payments by Medicare Advantage Plans

If you are covered by a Medicare Advantage program, the preceding discussion may or may not apply to you. Each Medicare Advantage carrier can negotiate payment contracts with each of its participating hospitals. Most MA plans have chosen to pay hospitals using the same method (i.e., DRGs) that Original Medicare uses, but some may apply their own methodologies. A Medicare Advantage plan is not obliged to reveal the content of a contract it has negotiated with a hospital, since such information is considered proprietary. Whatever the particular payment arrangement, you can count on the fact that the hospital will be trying its best to be efficient and cost effective, just as it does with Original Medicare patients. Under Medicare rules, if you are taken on an emergency basis to a hospital that doesn't participate with your Medicare Advantage plan, the hospital will be paid according to the DRG system, just as if you were insured by Original Medicare.

Admission versus Observation

Robert Davis was taken by ambulance to the emergency room because of chest pain that began at 1:00 AM. While out with friends that evening, he ate and drank more than usual. He's examined by the emergency room physician; blood tests and an electrocardiogram are done. There's concern that he's had a heart attack, but so far the tests are all negative. It's certainly not safe to send him home, so he's brought into the hospital. By the next afternoon he feels well and all tests for a heart attack remain negative. The pain was probably due to what he ate and drank. He goes home.

Was Robert admitted to the hospital? He was transferred to a room on a hospital floor, where he ended up staying overnight. Nurses checked him regularly, and he had continuous heart monitoring. But the answer is no. His stay in the hospital was not technically an admission. Rather it was classified as **observation,** which Medicare considers outpatient care.

Since the presumptive diagnosis was heart attack, the hospital should technically be paid according to the DRG for a heart attack. But Robert really didn't have one, and he went home the next day. The DRG for treatment of a heart attack would pay the hospital for substantially more services than he actually required and received. CMS has found this situation unacceptably costly.

For a patient's hospital stay to be officially considered an admission, a physician must specifically write an order that he be admitted. Until that order is written, the patient is still under observation. He's an outpatient and DRG payments do not apply. Why is this important to you? If the medical care is the same, why worry about how Medicare classifies your hospital stay?

⚠ **Your total cost sharing responsibility for an outpatient stay in the hospital (observation) can far exceed your expenses if you're an inpatient (admission), even though the outpatient stay is likely to be much shorter.**

Medicare Part B requires cost sharing on your part for *each of the separate services you receive for outpatient care,* including observation in a hospital. There will be a copay for the emergency room (up to $1,216 for this service alone), a copay for each test, and cost sharing for the hospital room as well. These can add up rapidly. This may seem unfair. You're right, it is. Unfortunately, it's a consequence of the different cost sharing provisions of Medicare Part A and Medicare Part B. What can you do about it?

First, you can make sure you have insurance that supplements Medicare. Even a Medigap Plan A (the least comprehensive one), which does not cover the Medicare Part A hospital deductible and therefore would leave you owing $1,216 for a short inpatient admission, does cover Medicare Part B coinsurance and copays.

Second, any time you find yourself in a hospital, make sure you specifically ask whether you have been admitted or are being observed. It will not necessarily be obvious. You should be informed of your status by a hospital representative, but in all the excitement of your illness and treatment, you may be unaware that someone has discussed what, at the time, seemed like a technicality. Inquire if you're unsure. Ask to speak to a hospital representative if you have questions.

It will be particularly important to know whether you've been classified as under observation for some period before finally being admitted, and you subsequently need post-hospital care at a skilled nursing facility.

Often a patient is initially classified as under observation and subsequently officially admitted when it becomes clear that admission is appropriate. When this occurs, the entire hospital stay is considered as an admission for payment by Medicare. It's covered solely by Medicare Part A, and you pay only a single Medicare Part A deductible. Unfortunately, when a hospital stay begins with observation, the entire stay does *not* count toward the three-day hospital *admission* requirement for Medicare to pay for subsequent SNF care. Logical? I will talk more about this when we discuss post-hospital care in the next chapter.

⚠ While less common, it's also possible for your status to change from admission to observation (when it's determined that you really didn't have the condition for which you were initially admitted). In this circumstance, Medicare Part B coverage and coinsurance will apply to the entire time you were in the hospital. Again, Medigap insurance can be a lifesaver.

So who makes all these critical observation-versus-admission decisions? The medical determinations will be made by your doctor with help from experts in Medicare compliance. One person essential to the process is someone you may never have heard of—she's the **case manager.**

Case Managers

Most case managers—also called **care coordinators, care managers,** or **discharge planners**—are RNs (some are social workers), but they'll never give you an injection or a pill, never change a dressing, and never restart your IV. Rather, they are the ones who guide you through the morass of insurance regulations, requirements, and discharge planning. They make sure the reason you're in the hospital and your subsequent hospital stay comply with the strict guidelines established by Medicare and other insurance carriers. Additionally, they work with you, your family, and your doctor(s) to implement planning your post-hospitalization care.

A CASE MANAGER IS **NOT** THE SAME PERSON THAT MANY HOSPITALS THESE DAYS CALL A "PATIENT CARE MANAGER." THE LATTER REFERS TO WHAT HAS TRADITIONALLY BEEN CALLED A "HEAD NURSE," WHO *DOES* PROVIDE AND SUPERVISE HANDS-ON CARE. WHETHER IT'S A HOSPITAL FLOOR, A SURGICAL SUITE, OR A RECOVERY ROOM, THE PATIENT CARE MANAGER IS THE RN RUNNING THE SHOW. PERSONALLY, I STILL PREFER THE TERM HEAD NURSE, BUT TODAY EVERYONE IS A MANAGER, SO KEEP THIS DISTINCTION IN MIND.

Leaving the Hospital

Starting several days before the planned date of discharge, the case manager begins to meet with the patient's physician to discuss post-discharge needs. Additionally, there are meetings with the patient himself and the patient's family, if appropriate. Using input from all these sources, a discharge plan is formulated. A whole slew of factors need to be considered, including the availability of family or friends to help, geographic distances, specific post-discharge therapeutic needs, other complicating medical conditions, finances, and the availability of services in the community. At times, patients object to how rapidly they are being discharged. Sometimes family members are similarly unhappy, out of either true medical concerns or the impact of the discharge on their own schedules. In general, case managers/discharge planners are quite expert at creating post-hospital plans that encompass both the medical and logistical needs of each patient. Some patients may not need more assistance than can be handled by family members. Others may be okay living at home but require additional services from nurses or therapists who provide specialized home care. Yet others may need continued inpatient care in a skilled nursing facility.

If a patient believes that he is being discharged from the hospital too soon, Medicare provides a specific appeals process using a local Quality Improvement Organization (QIO), which is not affiliated with the hospital and is charged by Medicare with making independent evaluations and rulings. The appeal can be requested anytime, including the proposed day of discharge, and the QIO must make its determination within 24 hours. Even if the QIO rules against the appeal, the patient is not responsible for paying for the one additional hospital day.

> THE RULES REGARDING APPEALS ARE OUTLINED IN A DOCUMENT ENTITLED "AN IMPORTANT MESSAGE FROM MEDICARE ABOUT YOUR RIGHTS," WHICH EVERY MEDICARE PATIENT SHOULD RECEIVE WITHIN TWO DAYS OF HOSPITALIZATION. IT DESCRIBES THE STEPS AND PROCEDURES OF A QIO REVIEW.

⚠️ *Think hard before you turn down post-discharge continuing care,* either inpatient care in an SNF or at home through a home care agency. Sure, you might feel you're okay and can go it alone. Perhaps you don't want to be away from home any longer. Or perhaps you've heard all kinds of horrible things about "being in a nursing home" and want nothing to do with a place like that. Medicare has strict requirements regarding acceptable post-hospitalization services, so the case manager obviously feels this care is justifiable under CMS's rules. Clearly your physician also thinks it will be helpful, and if you have any doubts, you can ask him why he thinks it's important. The additional care represents a valuable benefit for you. Be it intravenous antibiotics, physical therapy, or any other type of ongoing treatment, it may well speed your recovery or prevent a return to the hospital.

Choosing a Hospital

Patients enter the hospital through one of two routes: either through the emergency room (ER) or as scheduled admissions. Most planned admissions are for elective surgery or for medical therapy too toxic to be done as an outpatient. Rarely are people admitted to the hospital for *evaluations*—it's too expensive to hospitalize patients just for tests.

Sometimes you'll be able to select which hospital you'll be entering, and sometimes you won't. If there's only one hospital in your community, there are clearly no options. For planned major surgery or treatment of an unusual disease you might choose to travel to a medical center at some distance from your home, but for the most part you'll be using a local hospital.

In an emergency, an ambulance is likely to take you to the closest appropriate hospital for your condition. If you live in an urban area with multiple hospitals, you *might* be able to request a certain one. Whether that request will be honored will depend on the nature of your problem and how the emergency ambulance system works in your area. In life-threatening situations where every second counts, you will almost assuredly be rushed to the closest hospital that can handle your injury or illness. Driving an extra 15 minutes to reach your desired hospital will likely be considered dangerous, and they won't do it. In a less acute emergency, whether your choice will be honored will depend on the rules governing the local emergency medical service (EMS), which will vary by locale. If you live in an area with several available hospitals and you prefer one, learn about the local regulations ahead of time—when you're feeling fine. Check with your hospital or the agency that will be called when you dial 911. Don't wait until you're in the ambulance to find out!

For scheduled admissions, there still may be limitations on your choices. For example, there could be only a single hospital in your area equipped to perform a particular procedures. Or your surgeon might operate at only one hospital. If you are covered by Original Medicare, you may use any hospital that accepts Medicare, but if you have a Medicare Advantage plan your choices might be restricted. Your MA plan may only contract with certain specific hospitals in your area:

> *Bill Kuroda was on his way across town to a new hospital where he'd be having his second hip replacement. Four years ago Dr. Waldring had operated on the right one, and it was great. Now the left needed to be done too—but he had to go to a different hospital. "Sure is strange," Bill thought, "that Dr. Waldring is in my Medicare Advantage plan's provider panel, but a hospital where he operates isn't. Oh, well, I sure am glad that I checked before I scheduled the surgery there. I would have had no coverage at all! I suppose if Dr. Waldring operates at both hospitals, he must think both are okay."*

As for Bill, going outside an in-network hospital could result in no coverage or significant extra costs to you, depending on the details of your plan. Of course, in an emergency your MA plan must cover you in any hospital. But for elective admissions you'll have to be careful. Just because your doctor is an in-network provider and has staff privileges at a particular hospital does *not* mean the hospital is necessarily in-network. This is especially important with elective surgery. Make absolutely sure you establish the status of the hospital where you'll be treated.

EVALUATING HOSPITAL QUALITY

If you do have a choice of hospitals, there are some objective ways to compare them, and happily, Medicare itself is the source of one of them.

1. The Leapfrog Group is a nonprofit organization dedicated to promoting hospital safety and decreasing hospital errors. It's made up of prominent academic physicians who study ways to make hospitals safer. Using 26 criteria, they have created a Hospital Safety Score and used it to rate hospitals across the country. Each hospital gets a letter grade—either A, B, C, D, or F—depending on how they rate on several measures of patient safety that include rates of medical errors and adherence to recommended standards of practice. You can go to the website, www.hospitalsafetyscore.com, to see Leapfrog's methodology and to check on the scores received by hospitals that you are considering. The use of this website is free. These ratings are very helpful, but a couple of caveats. First of all, they measure only patient safety, not how good the hospital is at treating complicated medical conditions or simply getting patients better. Some community hospitals may have good safety scores, but they are not equipped to handle complex medical problems. Second, you need to interpret these ratings in the context of everything else you know about the hospital. The Leapfrog Group's rating criteria are stringent, meaning that getting an A is very difficult; many major, well-respected medical centers have C ratings.

2. CMS itself has created a useful tool for evaluating hospitals. You can access it at: www.hospitalcompare.hhs.gov. It provides extensive data on 4,000+ Medicare-certified hospitals throughout the country. There's a lot of information on the site, but it's most useful in allowing you to compare hospitals (three at a time) in your area. First enter your zip code; then pick three hospitals from the list of institutions. Click on the tab entitled **Patient Survey Results**. You'll be able to compare what patients felt about each of the hospitals on a variety of issues, such as how well doctors and nurses communicated with them, how promptly they received help or pain medication, overall cleanliness, and how well they received information on what

to do at home after discharge. Additionally, there are ratings on what percentage of patients gave the hospital a score of 9 or 10 (out of 10) and what percentage would *definitely* recommend the hospital to a friend. If you like, you can expand your choices and compare more hospitals. It's a helpful tool and, since it's provided by CMS, it's free.

3. The magazine *Consumer Reports,* an independent consumer publication that reviews many products and services and accepts no advertising, recently rated hospitals on a variety of factors including overall safety, bloodstream infections, avoiding readmissions, serious complications, overall patient experience, and hospital practices. An overall score of 1–100 was then given to each of the rated hospitals. Scores can be compared by selecting up to five hospitals from a given state or region. This information is available only to subscribers to their website, which is www.consumerreports.org.

In August, 2013, *Consumer Reports* released the results of a different hospital rating study. This one looked at surgical outcomes using data on Medicare patients at 2,463 U.S. hospitals, which were rated for five specific procedures and for overall results of all types of surgery. Results were controversial and sometimes startling, with nationally recognized medical centers often ranking poorly. Large hospitals did not necessarily do better than small ones; urban and rural hospitals performed about equally. The complete rating, listed by state and including how each hospital ranked, can be found on the *Consumer Reports* website (by subscription).

Chapter 10

Post-hospital, Home, and Hospice Care

Lila Chang knew she was lucky. When she had fallen in her apartment, her daughter had found her very quickly, noticed her slurred speech, and called 911 immediately. In the ER, they had started clot-busting drugs right away, and it appeared that she was improving from her stroke. Her speech had returned, but she still had weakness and couldn't walk. She'd been here in the hospital for seven days, and physical therapy already had helped. Her case manager, Ms. Goodson, had been discussing Lila's situation with her doctor, trying to find the best post-hospital program for her—possibly a skilled nursing facility or extensive home care. But a better option was found: She would be transferred to the rehabilitation wing of the hospital, where she could receive an intensive therapy program.

As we've seen, hospital coverage under Medicare is comprehensive, but stays are often short. In Chapter 9 we talked about how Medicare's prospective payment system, which compensates a hospital based on the patient's admitting diagnosis and contemplated treatment, but not on the length of stay, has put tremendous pressure on hospitals to keep patients for as few days as possible. The obvious consequence is that patients often need continued treatment once they've been discharged.

> **SHORT HOSPITAL STAYS = THE NEED FOR MORE POST-DISCHARGE TREATMENT.**

This often entails much more than simply continuing to take pills or resting to regain strength. Frequently, a therapeutic program requiring multiple health care professionals must continue well after it's time to leave the hospital. This might include continued intravenous antibiotics, wound care, physical therapy, or some combination of them. Post-hospital care has become a significant part of Medicare's constellation of covered services. It can be provided in several settings—as continued inpatient treatment in an extended-care facility, at home, or as a series of outpatient visits.

Additionally, there are many ill patients who can benefit from outpatient service designed to keep them out of the hospital. Others with end-stage diseases can be helped greatly by palliative care at home.

Available services covered by Medicare can be classified as follows:

- Post-hospital admission to a skilled nursing facility or other inpatient facility

- Home care

- Outpatient care

- Hospice care

Each has its own goals and unique requirements for coverage by Medicare.

Post-hospital Inpatient Care

As you know, Original Medicare covers post-hospital inpatient care if it occurs immediately after a hospital admission of at least three days. Shorter admissions and periods of observation are excluded. A physician must certify that the continued care is medically necessary; specific goals and a treatment plan must be delineated. In most facilities, Medicare Part A pays 100% of its approved fee for the first 20 days; for the next 80 days the patient is responsible for copays of $152 per day; beyond 100 days, Medicare payments cease.

When you read information from Medicare, whether in printed publications or on the website, post-hospital inpatient care is generally referred to as "skilled nursing facility care." In fact, it's a bit more complicated. Continuing post-hospital care can be provided in different inpatient settings, depending on the individual's particular needs. The common denominator of all Medicare-approved facilities is that they provide active, ongoing therapeutic and/or rehabilitative programs. Medicare is very specific regarding the types of services that are covered. Merely providing a milieu for recuperation is insufficient to meet Medicare's criteria. The key term is **skilled care**, which CMS defines as "A type of health care given when you need skilled nursing or rehabilitation staff to manage, observe, and evaluate your care. Nursing, physical therapy, occupational therapy, and speech therapy are considered skilled care by Medicare." (http://www.medicare.gov/ Homehealthcompare/resources/glossary.aspx)

Skilled nursing care vs. custodial care:

It's important to understand that custodial nursing home stays—nonskilled care that provides support services for daily living and is not therapeutic—is NOT covered by Medicare. Long-term, custodial care is considered the responsibility of the individual. It may also be covered by state Medicaid programs, and many people today take out long-term care insurance policies in recognition of the high cost of such care.

SKILLED NURSING FACILITIES

Medicare considers a **skilled nursing facility (SNF)** to be one that can provide skilled care, as defined above, and is Medicare certified. Being registered or licensed in a particular state or jurisdiction is not enough. The facility must be specifically Medicare certified, which means that it meets defined Medicare criteria and accepts Medicare assignment. Most post-hospitalization inpatients are treated in SNFs, which are generally able to provide nursing care, rehabilitation, or combinations of both. Typical examples of medical needs requiring skilled nursing include pneumonia, urinary tract infection, intravenous medication therapy, need for oxygen, tracheotomy care, wound care, and behavioral changes. Rehabilitative services include physical therapy, occupational therapy (which, incidentally, means therapy to improve a person's ability to perform normal daily functions—not helping someone find a job), and speech therapy. They may be oriented toward goals such as speeding improvement from surgery, improving function after a debilitating accident, or facilitating recovery from a stroke.

Most SNF admissions are arranged by hospital case managers. Once decisions have been made regarding the date of the hospital discharge and the type of continuing care needed, the race is on to find an appropriate placement. The discharge planner usually fires off faxes to multiple facilities. Every local SNF cannot necessarily provide every type of therapeutic program, so choices may be limited. In general, a facility near one's home or a family member's home is desirable. Of course, certain SNFs have better reputations than others. The preference of the patient is considered, but in the end the availability of beds limits the options. Occasionally a hospital will agree to keep a patient for an extra day to wait for a particular space to open, but this might require some serious cajoling. Ultimately, placement is up to the patient, who has the right to refuse any particular SNF.

⚠ **Medicare will cover an SNF admission that commences up to 30 days after hospital discharge, so keep in mind that one option (if medically reasonable) is to go home for a few days until the desired SNF bed becomes available.**

Choosing Your SNF

A common misconception is that a skilled nursing facility and a nursing home are synonymous. They're not, although they frequently occupy the same building. The term *nursing home* actually includes several levels of nursing care, ranging from intensive skilled nursing to custodial care. When most people think of "living in a nursing home," they are picturing custodial care, as noted in the box on page 155, often called *long-term care,* in which the goal is maintaining comfort. In some facilities, SNF patients are located in different areas from long-term care patients, but in others it's not possible to maintain this separation. As a result, many Medicare recipients who qualify for post-hospital nursing or rehabilitative care are hesitant to accept it. They simply can't picture themselves residing in a nursing home, with all that implies. There is no great solution for this, but you will sometimes have a choice regarding SNFs. You or a family member can query administrators at various SNFs to find out what their policies are in this regard.

You can use an online tool to look at various SNFs in your area by going to: www.Medicare.gov/nursinghomecompare/search.html Unfortunately, the listings cover all types of nursing and rehabilitation facilities. You won't be able to tell what services are available in each facility and which of them are appropriate for your particular post-hospital needs. For that information, you'll have to rely on your case manager's expertise. You or a loved one can try to check out some of the various available options, but typically it's not possible given the time constraints of finding an appropriate placement. On the other hand, if you are having elective surgery of a type that necessitates a post-hospital SNF stay (for example, a total knee replacement), you'll have time to do some research and possibly even be able to schedule the surgery and a concomitant SNF admission ahead of time.

How Medicare Pays for SNF Care

Medicare pays a skilled nursing facility on a <u>per diem</u> basis according to exactly what is done for each patient each day. If a person is receiving rehabilitation services, the number of sessions and the total number of minutes per week must be reported. For nursing services, the level of care has to be specified based on the diagnoses, symptoms, and precisely what nursing care is being provided. If both rehabilitation and nursing are required, then all components of both must be included. All this data is inputted into Medicare software and a fee for each day determined. Additionally, the SNF must show that a patient undergoing rehabilitation is making gains and attaining the goals for which the SNF admission was intended (called "gains and goals").

⚠️ **Even if services are being supplied, if the patient is not improving in the anticipated way, the SNF cannot justify continued inpatient care and the patient will have to be discharged (or pay out-of-pocket). Similarly, if a patient is unwilling to participate in physical therapy or refuses certain treatments, the stay in the SNF may have to terminate. Medicare is very strict about this. Remaining in the SNF without effort and improvement generally results in denial of coverage.**

Sometimes a patient's family won't accept this. Consider the following rather common scenario:

> *An elderly patient in an SNF simply doesn't want to go to physical therapy—it's hard work and too much effort. But it's the sole reason that he's there. When the SNF administrator informs the family members that their father must be discharged, first they become angry—they'll have to take care of him themselves at home. Then they ask her to "Just tell Medicare that he does go to therapy and is improving."*

⚠️ **Misrepresenting that a patient is attending therapy sessions and progressing toward the established goals for being in the SNF is Medicare fraud. Any SNF administrator would be crazy to do it. <u>Don't ask her to.</u>**

Another area of misunderstanding involves the fact that Medicare Part A covers 100% of Medicare approved costs for the first 20 days of SNF care. To some people, this implies that they are <u>entitled</u> to a 20-day stay in an SNF. This is decidedly not the case. As noted above, each day in the SNF must be justified as to need and progress. The 20 days refers only to the period of 100% coverage before cost sharing applies; it has nothing to do with any preapproval for 20 days of care. It's amazing how many patients come to an SNF with the expectation that they'll be there for exactly 20 days—they want the 20 free days to recuperate but intend to leave when daily copays commence. What a surprise when they must leave after seven or ten days because nothing more is being accomplished!

As a result of a recent class action lawsuit settlement (*Jimmo v. Sebelius*), there will be changes in CMS's regulations regarding the requirement for improvement to justify continued skilled care. Particularly for patients with chronic diseases that require such care to prevent deterioration of their conditions, the rules will be modified to allow continued skilled care (nursing or therapy) without need for actual improvement. This will not alter the 100-day limit, however, or affect cost sharing.

Under Original Medicare, when an individual no longer qualifies for SNF care, he or his representative must be given a "Skilled Nursing Facility Advanced Beneficiary Notice of Non-Coverage" at least one day prior to planned discharge. It explains why coverage will end, on what date, what out-of-pocket costs would apply if the patient stays, and how to file an appeal.

INPATIENT REHABILITATION FACILITIES

In some situations, patients require a rehabilitation program much more intensive than can be provided in most SNFs. These are often individuals who are generally in good health but have one problem that would benefit from an aggressive physical therapy approach They may need therapy following a severe accident such as a spinal cord injury or major orthopedic surgery such as a bilateral knee replacement. An option for such individuals is admission to an

inpatient rehabilitation facility (IRF), which may be a freestanding hospital devoted entirely to rehabilitation or a portion of an acute care hospital, such as a floor or wing, which similarly provides only rehabilitation. The minimum standards for such a facility are far more stringent than those for rehabilitation in an SNF. Each patient must be under the direct care of a rehabilitation physician who develops the therapeutic plan, supervises it, and personally sees the patient three times per week. Patients must be strong enough and motivated enough to handle the physical requirements of an intensive therapy protocol. It's not for everyone, but for the appropriate patient it can provide faster improvement. Additionally, IRFs have the ability to provide services that are simply too complex or specialized to be available in a typical SNF.

Medicare understands these differences and treats an inpatient rehabilitation facility as a hospital. In particular, Medicare does not pay an IRF by the day but according to a prospective payment system analogous to the DRG system used for acute care hospital admissions. In other words, the IRF receives a lump sum payment that depends on the condition being treated, the treatment plan, and additional medical problems potentially complicating the therapy. Patients are responsible for a one-time deductible of $1,216 (the same as for other hospital admissions). If a transfer occurs from an acute care hospital, there is no additional deductible. All the rules regarding benefit periods are identical to those for acute care hospital admissions.

> ONE SIGNIFICANT DIFFERENCE BETWEEN AN IRF AND AN SNF IS THAT MEDICARE WILL COVER DIRECT ADMISSIONS TO AN IRF. A PRIOR THREE-DAY ADMISSION TO ANOTHER HOSPITAL IS NOT REQUIRED.

Home Care

Many patients who leave the hospital don't want or really require treatment in an SNF, yet they do have continued medical needs that they cannot meet adequately by themselves. For some of these patients, Medicare provides coverage for home health services. Nursing care, rehabilitation, and various combinations of the two are available. All such services must be provided by a Medicare-certified home health agency. Even though these are outpatient in nature (that is, you're not in a hospital or an SNF), they are largely covered by Medicare Part A.

To qualify for home services under Medicare, three criteria have to be met. The patient must:

1. **Be homebound.** This means that she cannot leave the house for any substantial amount of time and, if she leaves, she does so primarily for medical appointments. Leaving the house must be physically taxing; assistance from another person or a device such as a walker or wheelchair is often needed.

2. **Require skilled care,** meaning the care of a registered nurse or licensed therapist. The need for assistance with walking, dressing, bathing, or eating is insufficient, as is being confused or forgetful.

3. **Be under the ongoing care of a physician.**

At the time of admission to the home care program, a physician must certify that the patient requires and qualifies for home care and must approve the entire plan of care. Services available for inclusion are skilled nursing, physical therapy, speech therapy, occupational therapy, medical social work, and assistance by a home health aide. It should be noted that the patient must require one of the first three services (skilled nursing, physical therapy or speech therapy) to qualify, but the others can be included in the plan. Typically, more than one service is provided.

WHAT MAKES UP A HOME CARE PROGRAM?

Let's first look at skilled nursing to get a feel for what a typical home care program is like. The visiting nurse comes to the house approximately three times per week, although visits may be more frequent initially. She performs three major tasks:

1. She observes the patient and assesses his overall condition, as well as improvement or worsening over time.

2. She performs needed hands-on treatments, such as complicated wound care or dressing changes.

3. She "teaches and trains" the caregiver at home. The importance of this educational component cannot be overemphasized, since the RN is there only a few hours per week, but the caregiver is there all the time. Instruction on how to correctly turn

someone in bed, how to properly care for a wound, and how to administer medications is essential to maximizing the benefits of home care. Physical therapy and speech therapy require direct intervention by the therapists, but training the caregiver in techniques to enhance the therapy adds to its effectiveness.

What About the Role of the Home Health Aide?

This is by far the most misunderstood element of home care. A home health aide provides hands-on services, such as bathing and dressing the patient, assisting with ambulation, and aiding with exercise—and typically for only 1 ½ hours twice a week. A home health aide is *not* a companion. He is an active caregiver who—like the RN or therapist—is available for limited periods and only for specific tasks. It's amazing how often the patient's family members are surprised that the aide isn't there to help all day, every day.

The assistance of a full-time aide is simply *not* part of a Medicare-funded home health plan.

The *Jimmo v. Sibelius* settlement mentioned earlier will have a substantial impact on home care. Chronically ill patients who require skilled services to maintain their level of functioning will now qualify for long-term home care. Previously, they were denied these services by Medicare because they didn't meet the "improvement standard." Patients who fall into this category include those suffering from ALS, multiple sclerosis, chronic wounds, Parkinson's disease, and a variety of similar chronic diseases. Only a skilled care program will be covered.

CHOOSING A HOME HEALTH AGENCY

If you are about to be discharged from a hospital and your physician has determined that home health care is appropriate, your case manager will send out a notice to local Medicare-approved home health agencies. Several or many will probably respond that they can provide the required services. You will then have a choice of providers. This is very different from trying to find an SNF with an available bed. Since you'll be at home, many agencies will be eager to treat you. How do you choose? A recommendation from your physician, the case manager, or a friend who has used a particular provider is a good place to start. Additionally, you can access a very useful tool on the Medicare website that will allow you to compare agencies. It's called *Home Health Compare*, and it's located at http://medicare.gov/homehealthcompare. Here's how to use it.

- On the first page of the website, enter your zip code and click *Search Agencies.*

- The next screen will show a list of local home care agencies and the services they provide. Now select any three of them by clicking the boxes to the left of their names, then clicking *Compare Now.*

- On the subsequent screen, above the names of the three agencies you've chosen, you'll see three tabs entitled *General Information, Quality of Patient Care,* and *Patient Survey Results.*

- Click on *Quality of Patient Care.* You'll see comparisons on a variety of measures. The most important ones—the ones that the agencies look at most carefully to see how they're stacking up—are the last two, which are how often their patients have to go to the emergency room and how often their patients require hospital admission. The lower the better!

- Now click on the tab entitled *Patient Survey Results.* Again, look at the last two items, which are measures of how happy patients have been with their care.

You can now do this for as many of the agencies as you like, but only three at a time.

> IT IS **NOT** NECESSARY TO HAVE A THREE-DAY HOSPITAL ADMISSION TO QUALIFY FOR HOME CARE SERVICES UNDER ORIGINAL MEDICARE. ALTHOUGH A SIGNIFICANT PROPORTION OF PATIENTS STARTING A HOME CARE PROGRAM DO COME DIRECTLY FROM A HOSPITAL, IT IS DEFINITELY NOT A REQUIREMENT FOR COVERAGE.

There are situations in which a doctor feels that a patient qualifies for, and would benefit from, skilled nursing care at home, often with the goal of preventing a hospital admission. This is a perfectly valid reason to commence home care. Remember, insurance companies, and this certainly includes Medicare, like nothing more than keeping their enrollees out of the hospital.

COVERAGE OF HOME HEALTH CARE BY ORIGINAL MEDICARE

As with hospitals, home health care agencies are compensated under Original Medicare using a prospective payment system. At the time a patient is initially assessed, information concerning diagnoses, functional level, and required services are obtained and used to determine how much Medicare will pay the agency for the first 60 days of treatment. This is a global fee that includes nursing visits, therapy, aides, social work, and any other services deemed necessary. At the end of the 60 days, a reassessment is made and payments adjusted based on changes in the patient's conditions or services actually provided. The agency receives one half of the total at the onset of the 60-day period and one half at the end, with adjustments up or down as appropriate. A physician must recertify any subsequent 60-day period, if needed. In actuality, although some patients require prolonged home care for problems such as nonhealing wounds, the average duration of home care treatment is presently about 35 days.

COVERAGE OF HOME HEALTH CARE BY MEDICARE ADVANTAGE PLANS

If you are covered by a Medicare Advantage plan, much of what was described above may not apply to you. Most Medicare Advantage plans handle home care differently than Original Medicare does. Many have contracts with specific home care agencies and therefore will not allow you to utilize any agency of your choice. You can still use the *Home Care Compare* tool described above, but you may have limited options to compare. Medicare Advantage plans may not employ a prospective payment system—they can pay by the day or by the service. The plan of care will have to be preapproved by the plan's medical director or staff, which can take time and delay treatment. Additionally, while an Original Medicare plan of care is initially approved for 60 days and then readjusted, an MA plan of care might be approved for a shorter period. Generalizing is difficult, since each MA plan will have its own rules regarding what constitutes a reasonable home care plan, how long it should last, and who will deliver the services. It is imperative that you check with your plan to learn its policies.

⚠ You can obtain many additional services from most home care agencies, but Medicare won't pay for them. Programs utilizing a variety of caregivers can be tailored to the needs of the individual— full-time companions, homemakers, private duty nurses, laundry and cleaning services, and meal preparation—and visits can be as frequent as desired; but all of it will have to be paid for privately.

Outpatient Care

Unfortunately, many individuals who would benefit greatly from home care don't qualify for it. In general, the most difficult criterion to meet is being homebound. If you can drive a car, even for a short distance, you don't qualify. If you regularly attend religious services or go to a senior center for activities, even with someone else driving, you probably won't qualify.

⚠ Homebound really means restricted to home with almost no outside travel.

Similarly, many people who would be helped by spending some time in an SNF cannot go to one, usually because they didn't have the required three-day hospital admission. If you don't meet the homebound criterion for home care and don't qualify for SNF care, all is not lost— there still are outpatient options available for completing your recovery. The cost of such services will be covered by Medicare Part B.

- Many hospitals now have wound care centers where continued therapy for surgical, traumatic, or pressure-related wounds can be provided. Typically, these centers can tailor therapeutic regimens to fit your ability to get to the center.

- Ongoing intravenous antibiotic therapy can be administered in many physicians' offices or hospital outpatient departments on a daily basis until the entire course has been completed.

- Physical therapy of all types, occupational therapy, and speech therapy are available in both freestanding and hospital-based physical therapy facilities.

When you're being discharged from the hospital, your doctor or the case manager can set you up with an appropriate provider that accepts your Medicare Part B coverage. *None of these services require a three-day hospital admission.*

Medicare Advantage plans will generally have specific in-network providers for outpatient rehabilitation and post-hospital care. You will have to check with your plan to see which ones are available to you and what approvals are needed to obtain these services.

Hospice Care

One of the greatest misconceptions in the field of medicine today is that hospice care provides only pain relief for terminally ill cancer patients. This idea distorts and vastly understates what hospice can accomplish for patients and their families. Certainly, the alleviation of pain is one of the objectives of hospice care, but there are many more. Most of you will be surprised to know that, nationwide, 62% of hospice patients do *not* have cancer[3]; they have a variety of other conditions ranging from neurological conditions such as ALS (Lou Gehrig's disease) to end-stage kidney failure to advanced Alzheimer's Disease. And for many in hospice, pain medications are not even part of their treatment programs. Hospice care is appropriate for anyone when there is no longer hope for cure or even improvement of a life-limiting illness and when the goal is living with dignity and without discomfort.

If hospice is not solely pain relief, what is it? Hospice care is an overall approach to providing comfort and support for terminally ill patients. It does not attempt to cure the underlying disease, but rather provides palliative treatment designed to keep the patient comfortable. Quality of life is paramount.

A major objective is allowing the patient to live out her life at home. A family member is commonly the primary caregiver. Hospice provides assistance and support, using a team approach that includes registered nurses, home health aides, social workers, clergy, and bereavement counselors. Medications are employed as appropriate for symptomatic relief. Treating such distressing symptoms as continual cough, persistent hiccups, confusion, or depression may be just as helpful as

[3] NHPCO Facts and Figures: Hospice Care in America. Alexandria, VA: National Hospice and Palliative Care Organization, October 2012, p. 7.

treating pain. Simple interventions like supplying oxygen to alleviate shortness of breath can provide amazing relief. Intravenous hydration and tube feeding, however, are not allowed. Many services are oriented toward helping family members cope with the difficulties involved with caring for their loved one, both physical and emotional. Additionally, bereavement counseling may continue for many months after the patient has passed on.

Most patients enter hospice at the suggestion of a physician or possibly a hospital case manager, although some insightfully raise the issue themselves. It's always a difficult subject to bring up. For some people, the word *hospice* carries negative connotations. They won't discuss entering hospice, but are willing to talk about forgoing continued attempts at curative measures and accepting a program of palliative or comfort care—which, of course, is exactly what hospice is all about.

> MEDICARE PART A PROVIDES ALMOST TOTAL COVERAGE FOR
> HOSPICE CARE; COST SHARING IS INSIGNIFICANT.

Medicare requires that several criteria be met. The attending physician and the hospice medical director must certify that the patient has a terminal illness and is unlikely to live for more than six months. The individual must agree to palliative care rather than further attempts at curative therapy and must sign a statement choosing hospice. All care must be provided by a Medicare-approved hospice program. If, while in hospice, a patient develops an unrelated medical problem that requires treatment, then Medicare Parts A & B cover that event (an example being a fall resulting in a fractured hip).

⚠ **The relationship between Medicare Advantage plans and hospice is unique. Any patient enrolled in a Medicare Advantage plan who qualifies for and elects hospice is immediately shifted to Original Medicare and ceases to be enrolled in the Medicare Advantage plan. As a result, there are no hospice patients in any MA plans.**

The decision to enter hospice is not irrevocable. Should a patient's medical condition improve and he wishes to withdraw from hospice, he can do so at any time; Original Medicare coverage then resumes. In fact, patients can actually "graduate" out of hospice. Sometimes the intensive supportive care provided by a hospice program is so effective that the patient's condition improves significantly. Ironically, he may no longer qualify for hospice care, since Medicare requires that there be symptoms to treat and that overall health be declining. (Examples of this are individuals with severe heart failure or chronic lung disease.)

Medicare pays the approved hospice program a fixed daily amount to provide for all the patient's needs. This includes costs for staff physicians, registered nurses, home health aides, social workers, bereavement counselors, therapists, certain medications, and medical equipment such as hospital beds, walkers, commodes, and wound dressings. On entry into the program, the physical and emotional needs of the individual are assessed and a plan formulated. Appropriate medical equipment is brought to the home. Family and friends carry out most of the day-to-day care. Hospice staff members are there to help and instruct, but are present only intermittently. Volunteers trained by the hospice agency contribute as well; in fact, CMS regulations require that care by volunteers constitute at least 5% of the hospice-provided hours. Such care can be given in whatever place the patient calls home—house, apartment, assisted living facility, or nursing home.

Although hospice care is primarily home care, patients can occasionally be admitted for short-term stays to hospice-approved inpatient facilities. Such admissions can occur either because of an acute change in the patient's condition or to provide **respite care**. Respite care, in which the hospice patient can remain in the facility for up to five days, is designed to allow an exhausted caregiver time to rest and recover from the rigors of providing continuous care.

Many authorities on the subject of hospice feel that it is underused and that patients typically enter the programs much later than they should. The median hospice stay nationwide is only 19 days.[4] In other words, half of all hospice participants remain under hospice care for 19 days or less. Many reasons have been cited for this. Physicians tend to resist "giving up" on their patients. Similarly, patients don't want to lose hope. Indeed, some physicians and some patients will never view hospice as a reasonable alternative to fighting on. Nevertheless, there are others who accept the realities of their conditions and see hospice as a blessing. For them, it's readily available under Medicare.

---

[4] Ibid, p. 5.

Chapter 11

Using Your Medicare Wisely

Rosalie Saunders walked hesitantly into her local senior center. As she neared the front desk, Jackie, the receptionist, greeted her: "Mrs. Saunders, so nice to see you. You look a bit out of sorts. Are you OK?" "I don't know where to turn," Rosalie replied. "In the last six months I've had a lot of doctors' appointments and tests. Now I'm getting these letters from Medicare and my other insurance company. Some of them are five or six pages long with all this stuff about visits and tests and copayments. I don't know if I owe money or what. I want to pay my bills, but I can't figure these things out. Can anyone help?" "Those things can really get confusing, Mrs. Saunders. I'll call Randy Pearson. He's our resident expert on Medicare and helps people all the time. He'll figure it out." Rosalie was visibly relieved. This was the kind of medicine she needed now.

Understand Your Coverage

To use your Medicare insurance effectively, you must know exactly what coverage you actually have. This may sound silly, but it's not. After reading the first part of this book, you should understand all about Original Medicare, including its component parts, and about Medicare Advantage (Medicare Part C). If you have chosen Original Medicare, you will need to present your red, white, and blue Medicare card plus your Medigap card every time you see a doctor, go to a laboratory, or have any type of service at a hospital. With a Medicare Advantage plan, you'll have a single card that's totally different (with a different number) from a regular Medicare card. You'd be shocked by how many people who have enrolled in a Medicare Advantage program present a regular Medicare card when they arrive at a doctor's office. It won't work! Medicare Drug plans will have a separate card under Original Medicare, but drug coverage under a Medicare Advantage plan may utilize the single card used for doctors, hospitals, and the like.

⚠️ **If you have Original Medicare, you might want to find a place to carry your Medicare card other than your wallet. This will be easier for women, who often have a handbag, than men. If your wallet is stolen and your Medicare card is in it, the thief will have access to not only your identification and credit cards but also your Social Security number, which is the number CMS uses as your ID number. This is a recipe for identity theft.**

Ironically, a number of years ago the federal government mandated that private insurance companies could no longer use Social Security numbers as ID numbers on medical insurance cards—specifically to help prevent identity theft. Yet CMS continues to use them. Logical? Some experts suggest you not carry your Medicare card with you, but you'll have lots of trouble if you see a new doctor or end up in an emergency room. If at all possible, carry your Medicare card with you, but separate from your wallet.

Paying Your Providers: Original Medicare

As you know, some physicians agree to accept Medicare assignment and others don't. A doctor who accepts Medicare assignment—a participating provider—agrees that Medicare's approved fee will serve as his full fee. Medicare will pay 80% of that fee and you will be responsible for the other 20%. With most Medigap plans, the insurance company will cover the 20%. A participating doctor will always send an electronic claim directly to Medicare. If you don't have a Medigap plan, you might be asked to pay the 20% at the time of your visit. With a Medigap plan, in most cases you will never be billed. Medicare will pay the doctor its 80% and then electronically forward the bill for the remaining 20% directly to the Medigap carrier. It's called "piggybacking" a claim, and it's great for you—you never have to deal with any paperwork. (It's more complicated if you have a Medigap plan K, L, N or high-deductible F, all of which employ partial payments or deductibles. So you'll need to learn the rules that go with them.) If your Medicare Part B coverage is supplemented by a private insurance policy, such as a small group employee insurance plan or a retirement plan from a former employer, you will probably have to pay the 20% yourself and then submit the claim on your own. Piggybacking often won't apply.

If your doctor doesn't accept assignment (he's non-participating), the maximum amount he can charge you will be Medicare's limiting fee, the calculation of which was discussed in detail in Chapter 3. He's required to send the claim directly to Medicare on your behalf, but he may expect full payment of the limiting fee at the time of the visit. If so, you will be reimbursed by Medicare for its portion of the bill. Some doctors may agree to have the Medicare payment sent directly to them, so you won't have to pay that portion of the bill, but doctors are under no obligation to do so. In any case, you will always have to pay the difference between Medicare's share and the limiting fee. No Medigap policies except F and G pay any portion of a bill from a non-participating provider. However, Medigap Plans F and G pay 100% of the difference between what Medicare pays and the limiting fee. Consequently, for patients with these plans, many doctors will bill Medicare directly with the remainder of the claim being piggybacked to the Medigap carrier.

The bottom line:

▶ *For a participating provider:* The most you might have to pay is 20% of the Medicare-approved fee, but nothing if you have most Medigap plans.

▶ *For a non-participating provider:* If you have a Medigap Plan F or G, you're completely covered. Otherwise, you must pay the difference between Medicare's portion and the limiting fee. You can be expected to pay the entire bill at the time of service, with a partial reimbursement from Medicare to follow, paid directly to you.

⚠ **I can't say it often enough: When you make a doctor's appointment or schedule a procedure, ask whether the provider is participating or non-participating.**

Paying Your Providers: Medicare Advantage

If your Medicare coverage is from a Medicare Advantage plan, the situation is quite different. Here every provider is either in-network or out-of-network. Your plan's fee schedule will determine how much of the cost of a particular service will be your responsibility. As you know, HMO-type plans can have very stringent restrictions on which doctors you can see and which hospitals you can use, while PPOs or point-of-service plans generally allow more flexibility. For any given service at any given provider, you might have a copay, coinsurance, or no coverage at all. You will be expected to pay your portion at the time of the visit; or you may have to pay the doctor's full fee if your plan doesn't cover her.

You may be very familiar with your plan's rules, but unsure of a particular physician's status. Ask her staff when you schedule an appointment, *not* when you arrive to be seen. If you feel the office staff doesn't understand what you're asking (a decided possibility), call your plan to establish with certainty the extent to which your visit with that provider will be covered. And always be sure to get the name of the person you talked to.

⚠ **Remember that providers include not just the doctor you're seeing but also the facility and any other professionals involved in the service you're getting. As explained in Chapter 6, your surgeon may be in-network but the surgicenter that's convenient for you and the anesthesiologist may not. Or when you have a diagnostic test like a colonoscopy, the gastroenterologist might be in-network, but perhaps the hospital is not. Similarly, make sure that any laboratory that your doctor uses is in-network. The moral: Be certain that you know whether every provider you'll be using is part of your plan's network.**

Advanced Beneficiary Notice of Noncoverage (ABN)

When there is doubt about whether Original Medicare will pay for a particular service, the provider will normally ask you to sign an **Advance Beneficiary Notice of Noncoverage (ABN)**. Signing this form acknowledges that you have been informed that you will have to pay for the service if Medicare does not. A copy of the official ABN form is shown on page 175. Look at it carefully. It's extremely important that you understand the implications of signing this form before you even consider doing so.

The upper half of the ABN lists your name and Medicare number, along with the service in question, the reason it might not be covered by Medicare, and the estimated cost. In the lower half, one of three options must be selected:

- **OPTION 1** is typically used when a particular service is often covered by Medicare but there are circumstances that, in your case, might make Medicare balk. Examples of this are diagnostic procedures for which Medicare restricts how often you can have them, such as mammograms, bone density studies, or colonoscopies. Let's say you've been diagnosed with osteoporosis on a previous bone density exam and are on drug therapy. Your doctor wants to check for effectiveness after one year—basically to determine whether it's worth continuing. Medicare typically pays for these studies only every two years. With a good explanation from your doctor CMS probably will pay, but because it's uncertain, you're being asked to sign the ABN. Some providers will require you to pay up front and then have your payment refunded if Medicare pays. Others will wait for Medicare's ruling. It may depend on how likely it is that Medicare will pay.

- **OPTION 2** most often applies to procedures that are cosmetic or discretionary. In this situation, you want the procedure and agree to pay for it. A good example is removal of a benign skin growth because you don't like its appearance. The service is considered "not medically necessary." Medicare is out of the payment loop but still requires documentation that you were informed by the physician that Medicare won't pay.

- **OPTION 3** is rarely used. It says you don't want the procedure.

⚠ **Pay special attention to the box entitled "(F) Estimated Cost," because it will determine how much you have to pay, and if OPTION 1 has been checked, that amount might be negotiable.**

If OPTION 2 has been checked, then the amount in box (F) will be the amount you agree to pay for the service. In the example given, you might have agreed to pay $125 to remove the skin growth.

But if it's OPTION 1, the amount is not so clear, since there are *two* possible fees. Every provider has a regular fee for every service, but there's also a Medicare-approved fee. If Medicare agrees to pay the claim, then the provider receives the Medicare-approved fee as full payment (less any coinsurance or copay). *But most providers will put their regular fees in box (F), and the differences between regular and Medicare-approved fees can be substantial.* In the bone density example above, the regular fee could be $650 and the Medicare-approved fee $225. *Yes, the differences are frequently that great.* **I believe you have a perfect right to request that the fee you will have to pay be the same as the Medicare-approved fee.** Why, you should ask, should you pay $650 if the claim is denied, when the provider is willing to accept $225 if Medicare agrees to pay? What incentive does the provider have to push Medicare to pay the claim if payment from you will be so much greater? You may not be successful in getting the provider to agree to the lower amount, but you never know. You might be surprised. Be knowledgeable, logical, and persistent. Always try.

(A) Notifier(s):
(B) Patient Name: *(C)* Identification Number:

ADVANCE BENEFICIARY NOTICE OF NONCOVERAGE (ABN)

NOTE: If Medicare doesn't pay for *(D)*_____ below, you may have to pay.

Medicare does not pay for everything, even some care that you or your health care provider have good reason to think you need. We expect Medicare may not pay for the *(D)*_____ below.

*(D)*_____	*(E)* Reason Medicare May Not Pay:	*(F)* Estimated Cost:

WHAT YOU NEED TO DO NOW:

- Read this notice, so you can make an informed decision about your care.
- Ask us any questions that you may have after you finish reading.
- Choose an option below about whether to receive the *(D)*_____ listed above.
  Note: If you choose Option 1 or 2, we may help you to use any other insurance that you might have, but Medicare cannot require us to do this.

(G) OPTIONS: Check only one box. We cannot choose a box for you.

❑ **OPTION 1.** I want the *(D)*_____ listed above. You may ask to be paid now, but I also want Medicare billed for an official decision on payment, which is sent to me on a Medicare Summary Notice (MSN). I understand that if Medicare doesn't pay, I am responsible for payment, but **I can appeal to Medicare** by following the directions on the MSN. If Medicare does pay, you will refund any payments I made to you, less co-pays or deductibles.

❑ **OPTION 2.** I want the *(D)*_____ listed above, but do not bill Medicare. You may ask to be paid now as I am responsible for payment. **I cannot appeal if Medicare is not billed.**

❑ **OPTION 3.** I don't want the *(D)*_____ listed above. I understand with this choice I am not responsible for payment, and **I cannot appeal to see if Medicare would pay.**

H) Additional Information:

This notice gives our opinion, not an official Medicare decision. If you have other questions on this notice or Medicare billing, call **1-800-MEDICARE** (1-800-633-4227/TTY: 1-877-486-2048). **Signing below means that you have received and understand this notice. You also receive a copy.**

(I) Signature:	*(J)* Date:

According to the Paperwork Reduction Act of 1995, no persons are required to respond to a collection of information unless it displays a valid OMB control number. The valid OMB control number for this information collection is 0938-0566. The time required to complete this information collection is estimated to average 7 minutes per response, including the time to review instructions, search existing data resources, gather the data needed, and complete and review the information collection. If you have comments concerning the accuracy of the time estimate or suggestions for improving this form, please write to: CMS, 7500 Security Boulevard, Attn: PRA Reports Clearance Officer, Baltimore, Maryland 21244-1850.

Form CMS-R-131 (03/08)   Form Approved OMB No. 0938-0566

The Importance of Record Keeping

As people age, they tend to need more and more medical services. Consequently, even relatively healthy seniors end up seeing quite a few different providers. They see their PCP and perhaps an ophthalmologist to manage glaucoma, a dermatologist to check a new skin growth, or a rheumatologist in consultation for unexplained joint pain. A fall might necessitate an emergency room visit. Perhaps it's time for a routine mammogram or a colonoscopy. And, of course, blood tests of all sorts require trips to the laboratory. For someone with significant medical problems, the number of visits increases dramatically. Every service you receive will have a bill of some type associated with it. Depending on your precise coverage, you may receive many bills or none at all. You may have to deal with deductibles, copays, coinsurance, or bills for the entire cost of a service. It can be confusing for almost everyone and overwhelming for those with lots of medical needs.

As a result, it is imperative that you keep a detailed record of every encounter you have with the health care system. You can do it on a computer or in a hand-written notebook. It doesn't matter what method you use, although I'd recommend against loose slips of paper that easily get lost. Keep the record chronologically. It's simple. Every time you have a doctor's appointment, enter the date, which doctor you saw, and what was done, including the office visit, tests, and procedures. You may or may not receive a bill at the time of service. If you do, record the amount of the charges, the amount you paid, and how you paid (check, credit card, or cash). Do the same for laboratories, physical therapy appointments, X-rays, diagnostic procedures—every time you receive any kind of medical service, enter the information as soon as you get home. Don't put it off. Similarly, whenever you fill a prescription, keep a record of that. Be sure to include prescriptions you receive by mail order.

The Importance of the Explanation of Benefits (EOB)

An **explanation of benefits** (commonly called simply an **EOB** in medical circles) is a written communication from an insurance carrier explaining what charges were submitted to it for payment, what payments were made, to whom they were paid, and the reason(s) for payment or denial of the claim. EOBs in varying formats are used by virtually every medical insurance company to provide information to both patients and providers. CMS is no different. For Original Medicare participants, CMS sends its version of an EOB—called a **Medicare Summary Notice**— to every patient for whom bills were received during a three-month period. These notices list every claim that was submitted, including the date, the provider, the services provided, and the billing codes associated with the services.

For physician visits, the following information will be shown:

- the name of the service and its code

- whether or not the service was approved

- the amount charged

- the amount Medicare approved

- the amount Medicare paid the provider or is paying you

- the maximum amount you can be billed by the provider

Notes will address any deductible, whether the claim was piggybacked to your Medigap carrier, and other information unique to the particular claim. For outpatient facilities, hospitals, and other types of providers, the exact information on the Medicare Summary Notice may be slightly different, but in all cases you should have enough information to basically understand how Medicare handled the claim. If Medicare is sending you a check, you may receive notices more frequently than quarterly.

When you have a Medigap plan, the insurance company will also send you EOBs on a regular basis. These will list information similar to what's on the Medicare Summary Notice, but will also include how much the Medigap carrier paid to the providers or is paying to you.

On the following pages you will see the EOBs that one patient received regarding medical office visits with two different physicians, as well as a series of radiology services. The first one is her Part B Medicare Summary Notice for physician services (on the first three pages), the second is her Part B Medicare Summary Notice for facility charges for the radiology services (the next two pages), and the third is the EOB from her Medigap Plan F insurance company that corresponds to both of the Medicare EOBs (the final three pages). They are actual EOBs but have been slightly modified to remove identifying information. Take some time to review them. Some of the entries might be confusing and some of Medicare's calculations might not seem to add up. After the final page of EOB's, I'll explain how to interpret and understand them.

Sample EOBs

Your Claims for Part B (Medical Insurance)

Part B Medical Insurance helps pay for doctors' services, diagnostic tests, ambulance services, and other health care services.

Definitions of Columns

Service Approved?: This column tells you if Medicare covered the service.

Amount Provider Charged: This is your provider's fee for this service.

Medicare-Approved Amount: This is the amount a provider can be paid for a Medicare service. It may be less than the actual amount the provider charged.

Your provider has agreed to accept this amount as full payment for covered services. Medicare usually pays 80% of the Medicare-approved amount.

Amount Medicare Paid: This is the amount Medicare paid your provider. This is usually 80% of the Medicare-approved amount.

Maximum You May Be Billed: This is the total amount the provider is allowed to bill you and can include a deductible, coinsurance, and other charges not covered. If you have Medicare Supplement Insurance (Medigap policy) or other insurance, it may pay all or part of this amount.

June 25, 2013

Service Provided & Billing Code	Service Approved?	Amount Provider Charged	Medicare- Approved Amount	Amount Medicare Paid	Maximum You May Be Billed	See Notes Below
Dr.						
Established patient office or other outpatient visit, typically 15 minutes (99213)	Yes	$110.00	$78.28	$37.30	$40.22	A,B,C
Total for Claim #02-13179		$110.00	$78.28	$37.30	**$40.22**	D

Continued →

Notes for Claims Above

A $30.70 of this approved amount has been applied toward your deductible.

B The approved amount is based on a special payment method.

C After your deductible and coinsurance were applied, the amount Medicare paid was reduced due to Federal, State and local rules.

D We have sent your claim to your Medigap insurer. Send any questions regarding your benefits to them. Your Medigap insurer is UNITEDHEALTH GROUP.

June 28, 2013

Service Provided & Billing Code	Service Approved?	Amount Provider Charged	Medicare-Approved Amount	Amount Medicare Paid	Maximum You May Be Billed	See Notes Below
New patient office or other outpatient visit, typically 60 minutes (99205)	Yes	$477.00	$218.09	$170.98	$43.62	E,F
Total for Claim #02-13191		$477.00	$218.09	$170.98	$43.62	G

June 28, 2013

Service Provided & Billing Code	Service Approved?	Amount Provider Charged	Medicare-Approved Amount	Amount Medicare Paid	Maximum You May Be Billed	See Notes Below
Ultrasound of breast (76645-26) professional charge	Yes	$125.00	$28.05	$21.99	$5.61	E,F
Claim #02-1318					(continued)	

Continued →

Notes for Claims Above

E The approved amount is based on a special payment method.

F After your deductible and coinsurance were applied, the amount Medicare paid was reduced due to Federal, State and local rules.

G We have sent your claim to your Medigap insurer. Send any questions regarding your benefits to them. Your Medigap insurer is

June 28, 2013 t continued...

Service Provided & Billing Code	Service Approved?	Amount Provider Charged	Medicare-Approved Amount	Amount Medicare Paid	Maximum You May Be Billed	See Notes Below
Diagnostic mammography, producing direct digital image, unilateral, all views (G0206-26) professional charge	Yes	70.00	36.64	28.72	7.33	H,I
Diagnostic x-ray (77051-26) professional charge	Yes	10.00	3.27	2.57	0.65	H,I
Total for Claim #02-13186–		$205.00	$67.96	$53.28	$13.59	J

July 10, 2013
Radiology

Service Provided & Billing Code	Service Approved?	Amount Provider Charged	Medicare-Approved Amount	Amount Medicare Paid	Maximum You May Be Billed	See Notes Below
Ultrasound of breast (76645-26) professional charge	Yes	$125.00	$28.05	$21.99	$5.61	H,I
Total for Claim #02-13197-		$125.00	$28.05	$21.99	$5.61	J

Notes for Claims Above

H The approved amount is based on a special payment method.

I After your deductible and coinsurance were applied, the amount Medicare paid was reduced due to Federal, State and local rules.

J We have sent your claim to your Medigap insurer. Send any questions regarding your benefits to them. Your Medigap insurer is

Your Outpatient Claims for Part B (Medical Insurance)

Part B Medical Insurance helps pay for outpatient care provided by certified medical facilities, such as hospital outpatient departments, renal dialysis facilities, and community health centers.

Definitions of Columns

Service Approved? This column tells you if Medicare covered the outpatient service.

Amount Facility Charged: This is your facility's fee for this service.

Medicare-Approved Amount: This is the amount a facility can be paid for a Medicare service. It may be less than the actual amount the facility charged. The facility has agreed to accept this amount as full payment for covered services. Medicare usually pays 80% of the Medicare-approved amount.

Amount Medicare Paid: This is the amount Medicare paid the facility. This is usually 80% of the Medicare-approved amount.

Maximum You May Be Billed: This is the total amount the facility is allowed to bill you and can include a deductible, coinsurance, and other charges not covered. If you have Medicare Supplement Insurance (Medigap policy) or other insurance, it may pay all or part of this amount.

June 28, 2013

Service Provided & Billing Code	Service Approved?	Amount Facility Charged	Medicare-Approved Amount	Amount Medicare Paid	Maximum You May Be Billed	See Notes Below
Diagnostic mammography, producing direct digital image, unilateral, all views (G0206)	Yes	$419.00	$419.00	$85.90	$21.91	
Computer analysis of diagnostic mammogram (77051)	Yes	89.00	89.00	6.25	1.59	
Ultrasound of breast (76645)	Yes	371.00	371.00	49.85	26.76	
Total for Claim #2131910		$879.00	$879.00	$142.00	$50.26	A,B

Continued →

Notes for Claims Above

A The amount Medicare paid the provider for this claim is $142.00.

B After your deductible and coinsurance were applied, the amount Medicare paid was reduced due to Federal, State and local rules.

July 10, 2013

Referred by

Service Provided & Billing Code	Service Approved?	Amount Facility Charged	Medicare- Approved Amount	Amount Medicare Paid	Maximum You May Be Billed	See Notes Below
Ultrasound of breast (76645)	Yes	$371.00	$371.00	$49.85	$26.76	
Total for Claim #2132030:		$371.00	$371.00	$49.85	$26.76	C,D

Notes for Claims Above

C The amount Medicare paid the provider for this claim is $49.85.

D After your deductible and coinsurance were applied, the amount Medicare paid was reduced due to Federal, State and local rules.

Plan Code & Service Date(s) Provider Type of Service	Amount Charged	Medicare Approved Amount	Applied to Medicare Deductible	Medicare Paid	Plan Cost-Share	Your Plan Paid	Items & Notes
F 06/25/13	110.00	78.28	30.70	38.06		9.52	Ⓐ
Doctor's office visit							
F 06/25/13						30.70	Ⓑ
Pt B deductible							
Totals	$110.00	$78.28	$30.70	$38.06		$40.22	

$0.00   Your plan paid to you
$40.22   Your plan paid to provider

Notes

Ⓐ Your Plan benefit was based on the Medicare Approved Amount because your provider accepted Medicare assignment.

Ⓑ Your Plan paid the amount that was applied to the Medicare Part B deductible on this claim.

Claim 32030-   **Claim Processed**
                                                    07/31/13

Plan Code & Service Date(s) Provider Type of Service	Amount Charged	Medicare Approved Amount	Applied to Medicare Deductible	Medicare Paid	Plan Cost-Share	Your Plan Paid	Items & Notes
F 06/28/13	879.00	879.00		828.74		50.26	Ⓐ
Mammogram to aid diagnosis							
Totals	$879.00	$879.00		$828.74		$50.26	

$0.00   Your plan paid to you
$50.26   Your plan paid to provider

Notes

Ⓐ Your Plan benefit was based on the Medicare Approved Amount because your provider accepted Medicare assignment.

Claim 32057-   **Claim Processed**
                                                    07/25/13

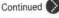
Continued

219AARPER1001001-06448-03

Page 4 of 6   Statement Date: August 7, 2013

Plan Code & Service Date(s) Provider Type of Service	Amount Charged	Medicare Approved Amount	Applied to Medicare Deductible	Medicare Paid	Plan Cost-Share	Your Plan Paid	Items & Notes
F 06/28/13	125.00	28.05		22.44		5.61	Ⓐ
Breast ultrasound							
F 06/28/13	70.00	36.64		29.31		7.33	Ⓐ
Mammogram to aid diagnosis							
F 06/28/13	10.00	3.27		2.62		0.65	Ⓐ
Physician review of mammogram							
Totals	$205.00	$67.96		$54.37		$13.59	

$0.00   Your plan paid to you
$13.59   Your plan paid to provider

Notes

Ⓐ Your Plan benefit was based on the Medicare Approved Amount because your provider accepted Medicare assignment.

Claim 32 100-4   **Claim Processed 07/30/13**

Plan Code & Service Date(s) Provider Type of Service	Amount Charged	Medicare Approved Amount	Applied to Medicare Deductible	Medicare Paid	Plan Cost-Share	Your Plan Paid	Items & Notes
F 06/28/13	477.00	218.09		174.47		43.62	Ⓐ
New doctor visit, 45+ minutes							
Totals	$477.00	$218.09		$174.47		$43.62	

$0.00   Your plan paid to you
$43.62   Your plan paid to provider

Continued ⏩

Notes

🅐 Your Plan benefit was based on the Medicare Approved Amount because your provider accepted Medicare assignment.

Claim 32140-ᶜ						**Claim Processed 08/06/13**	

Plan Code & Service Date(s) Provider Type of Service	Amount Charged	Medicare Approved Amount	Applied to Medicare Deductible	Medicare Paid	Plan Cost-Share	Your Plan Paid	Items & Notes
F 07/10/13	371.00	371.00		344.24		26.76	🅐
Breast ultrasound							
Totals	$371.00	$371.00		$344.24		$26.76	

$0.00   Your plan paid to you
$26.76 Your plan paid to provider

Notes

🅐 Your Plan benefit was based on the Medicare Approved Amount because your provider accepted Medicare assignment.

Claim 3214?						**Claim Processed 08/05/13**	

Plan Code & Service Date(s) Provider Type of Service	Amount Charged	Medicare Approved Amount	Applied to Medicare Deductible	Medicare Paid	Plan Cost-Share	Your Plan Paid	Items & Notes
F 07/10/13	125.00	28.05		22.44		5.61	🅐
Breast ultrasound							
Totals	$125.00	$28.05		$22.44		$5.61	

$0.00   Your plan paid to you
$5.61   Your plan paid to provider

Continued

Looking at the Medicare Summary Notices first, note the following:

- The Medicare-Approved Amount is often lower than the Amount Provider Charged in these examples, sometimes strikingly so, particularly for the radiology professional charges.

- For the second office visit (dated June 28, 2013) Medicare approved $218.09 and the patient was responsible for 20% of that, or $43.62 (the amount in the column entitled **Maximum You May Be Billed**). The provider was paid $170.98, which is a bit less than 80% of the approved amount (which would be $ 174.47). This relates to footnote **F** (described at the bottom of the page). You will often see footnotes like this; they do not affect the amount you must pay. Don't try to figure out why the physician or other provider is receiving less than 80% of the approved amount—you generally can't.

- For the first office visit (dated June 25, 2013) the physician received less than half of the amount Medicare approved. In this case, footnote **A** tells us that the patient had not met her Part B annual deductible (more specifically, she had $30.70 remaining on her deductible), so her cost sharing responsibility was higher, totaling $40.22. The amount the physician received from CMS was affected by both the deductible and the "special rules" footnote. *Always look at the footnotes—they're important!*

- For the two facility fees in the second Medicare Summary Notice (dated June 28, 2013 and July 10, 2013 on pages 182-183), you will note that the Amount Medicare Paid is *far* less than the amount it approved, but you will not be able to figure out why the facilities got so much less than the approved fee.

- These examples illustrate that the calculations can sometimes be complicated, but the critical number for you will always be the **Maximum You May Be Billed** column.

- Each of the services for this patient has a footnote stating that the claim was sent on to the Medigap insurer (i.e., it was piggybacked).

Now look at the EOB from the Medigap carrier. It covers exactly the same claims as the Medicare Summary Notices.

- All of the services listed in the two Medicare Summary Notices also appear on the Medigap EOB, although not necessarily in the same order. Additionally, services by the same provider are grouped differently. However, you should be able to match the corresponding services and payments on the Medicare and Medigap EOBs.

- In this group of EOBs, for every service, the amount under **Maximum You May Be Billed** is identical to the amount the Medigap carrier paid, as seen in the **Your Plan Paid** column.

- Since this patient chose to have a Medigap Plan F, her Medigap carrier paid all of her cost sharing, including the remaining part of her Part B deductible, coinsurance for her physician fees, and copays for the facility fees.

Obviously, all EOBs will not be the same, and many will be quite complicated, depending on how many different providers you've seen, whether or not they accept assignment, and the type of Medigap policy you have selected. Don't be afraid of them. EOBs are truly your best friend! They allow you to make sure you are being charged only for services you actually received. Look at them carefully. Check what you see listed on the EOBs against the list of services you believe you've received—the list discussed in the box **"The Importance of Record Keeping."**

If you are covered by a Medicare Advantage plan, you will also receive EOBs. They will come from the insurance company running the plan, not from CMS, but the principle of reconciling the services you actually received with what's shown on the EOBs remains the same.

EOB Information on the Internet

Everyone who has Original Medicare will get a Medicare Summary Notice for every three-month period in which any claims were filed. It will come automatically by U.S. mail. However, you might want to look at your claims more quickly. If you're comfortable with computers, there's a great way to do it. You can go to https://www.MyMedicare.gov and sign up to get Internet access to all your claims data. When you go to the website (actually, you can just type in mymedicare.gov), you'll be instructed on how to sign up. You'll have to enter your Medicare number (don't be afraid—it's a legitimate Medicare site!) and choose a username and password. It's simple to do and you will be registered immediately.

The site contains information about any claim filed on your behalf. Claims information appears quite quickly—often within a week or two. You can search old claims as well. The amount of detail is far greater than on the paper EOBs. If you like using the Internet, definitely get a MyMedicare.gov account and start exploring what's there. It's a great way to get a firm handle on all your Original Medicare claims. Using this site can be particularly helpful when EOBs from your Medigap carrier arrive *before* the Medicare Summary Notice arrives—which occurs routinely. You'll be able to reconcile the MyMedicare site's claims data with the Medigap EOBs.

If you have a Medicare Advantage plan, your claims information will *not* appear on the MyMedicare.gov website. However, your plan will most likely have a way for you to access claims data on the web. Some plans allow you to get your EOB's online. They send you an email when a new EOB is available and you can then click on a link or go to the website to look at the new posting. The formats of Medicare Advantage websites will vary, as will their ease of use. Check with your individual plan to see what online services are available and how to access them.

Medicare Drug Plan EOBs—Even More Information, Even More Complicated

Medicare Part D drug plans operate very differently from all other parts of Medicare. It doesn't matter whether they are separate Part D plans or ones that are incorporated into Medicare Advantage programs. Drug plan EOBs, called **Monthly Prescription Drug Summaries**, contain a great deal of information. The drug summary will indicate the amount the plan paid and the amount you paid for each prescription you filled during the month. The total amounts paid by the plan and by you during the month and year-to-date will also be shown. The EOB will then indicate what "drug payment stage" you're in. You may recall from our discussion of Part D plans that there are four payment stages. Stage One is the Yearly Deductible stage—you pay 100% of full price. During Stage Two—the Initial Coverage stage—you pay the plan's established fee for each drug, which will depend on its tier. Stage Three is the Coverage Gap (the donut hole), in which your expenses are much higher. In Stage Four—the Catastrophic Coverage stage—government subsidies markedly decrease your drug costs.

The EOB will tell you which stage you're presently in and how far you are from leaving that stage. Totals for "out-of-pocket costs" and "total drug costs" will also be shown. You'll need these to figure out when you might be changing stages. As you know, Medicare Part D is unnecessarily complicated, so the EOBs have to be complicated too. Even if you fill only one prescription in a particular month, the Monthly Prescription Drug Summary will be several pages long. Don't let that dissuade you from looking at it carefully and reconciling it with the medication list you have kept.

Let's look at a typical Medicare Drug Plan EOB (shown below) for someone who filled four prescriptions in one month. I have compressed multiple pages for clarity.

- Section 1 lists the prescriptions filled during the month, including name, strength, and amount. How much the plan paid and how much you paid (generally your copay, occasionally your coinsurance) for each are also shown, along with total costs for the month. Below that are totals year-to-date. It's pretty straightforward.

- Section 2 explains the four drug payment stages, indicates where you are in the progression, and lets you know what additional expenditures will move you into the next stage.

- Section 3 indicates your current "total drug costs" and "out-of-pocket costs," which are the values used to calculate when you enter and escape from the donut hole respectively.

Just as you should always check your EOBs against the records you've kept of your medical encounters, you should similarly reconcile your list of prescriptions you've filled with the drug plan EOBs.

Sample Medicare Drug Plan EOB

SECTION 1. Your prescriptions during the past month

- Chart 1 shows your prescriptions for covered Part D drugs for the past month.
- **Please look over this information about your prescriptions to be sure it is correct.** If you have any questions or think there is a mistake, Section 5 tells what you should do.

CHART 1. Your prescriptions for covered Part D drugs April 2012	Plan paid	You paid	Other payments (made by programs or organizations, see Section 3)
Zolpidem Tab 10mg 04/20/2012 Pharmacy Rx# 00000431 30 Days Supply	$0.00	$5.49	
Pantoprazole Tab 40mg 04/24/2012 Rx# 00007534 90 Days Supply	$59.75	$8.00	
Amlodipine Tab 10mg 04/24/2012 Rx# 0000753 90 Days Supply	$9.17	$0.00	
Atorvastatin Tab 40mg 04/24/2012 Rx# 0000764 90 Days Supply	$253.07	$117.00	
TOTALS for the month of April 2012: **Your "out-of-pocket costs" amount is $130.49.** (This is the amount you paid this month ($130.49) plus the amount of "other payments" made this month that count toward your "out-of-pocket costs" ($0.00). See definitions in Section 3.) **Your "total drug costs" amount is $452.48.** (This is the total for this month of all payments made for your drugs by the plan ($321.99) and you ($130.49) plus "other payments" ($0.00).)	$321.99 (total for the month)	$130.49 (total for the month) (Of this amount, $130.49 counts toward your out-of-pocket costs.)	$0.00 (total for the month)
Year-to-date totals **01/01/2012 through 04/30/2012**	Plan paid	You paid	Other payments (made by programs or organizations, see Section 3)
Your year-to-date amount for "out-of-pocket costs" is $297.76. **Your year-to-date amount for "total drug costs" is $907.50.** For more about "out-of-pocket costs" and "total drug costs," see Section 3.	$609.74 (year-to-date total)	$297.76 (year-to-date total) (Of this amount, $297.76 counts toward your out-of-pocket costs.)	$0.00 (year-to-date total)

SECTION 2. Which "drug payment stage" are you in?

As shown below, your prescription drug coverage has "drug payment stages." How much you pay for a prescription depends on which payment stage you are in when you fill it. During the calendar year, whether you move from one payment stage to the next depends on how much is spent for your drugs.

	You are in this stage:		
STAGE 1 **Yearly Deductible**	**STAGE 2** **Initial Coverage**	**STAGE 3** **Coverage Gap**	**STAGE 4** **Catastrophic Coverage**
• (Because there is no deductible for the plan, this payment stage does not apply to you.)	• You begin in this payment stage when you fill your first prescription of the year. During this payment stage, the plan pays its share of the cost of your drugs and you (or others on your behalf) pay your share of the cost.	• During this payment stage, you (or others on your behalf) receive a discount on brand name drugs and you pay only 86% of the costs of generic drugs. • You generally stay in this stage until the amount of your year-to-date "out-of-pocket costs" (see Section 3) reaches $4,700. When this happens, you move to stage 4, Catastrophic Coverage.	• During this payment stage, the plan pays most of the cost for your covered drugs. • You generally stay in this stage for the rest of the calendar year (through December 31, 2012).

What happens next?

Once you have **an additional $2,022.50 in "total drug costs,"** you move to the next payment stage (stage 3, Coverage Gap).

SECTION 3. Your "out-of-pocket costs" and "total drug costs" (amounts and definitions)

We're including this section to help you keep track of your "out-of-pocket costs" and "total drug costs" because these costs determine which drug payment stage you are in. As explained in Section 2, the payment stage you are in determines how much you pay for your prescriptions.

Your "out-of-pocket costs"	**Your "total drug costs"**
$130.49 month of April 2012	$452.48 month of April 2012
$297.76 year-to-date (since January 2012)	$907.50 year-to-date (since January 2012)

DEFINITION:

"Out-of-pocket costs" includes:

- What you pay when you fill or refill a prescription for a covered Part D drug. (This includes payments for your drugs, if any, that are made by family or friends.)
- Payments made for your drugs by any of the following programs or organizations: "Extra Help" from Medicare; Medicare's Coverage Gap Discount Program; Indian Health Service; AIDS drug assistance programs; most charities; and most State Pharmaceutical Assistance Programs (SPAPs).

It does not include:

- Payments made for: a) plan premiums, b) drugs not covered by our plan, c) non-Part D drugs (such as drugs you receive during a hospital stay), d) drugs obtained at a non-network pharmacy that does not meet our out-of-network pharmacy access policy.
- Payments made for your drugs by any of the following programs or organizations: employer or union health plans; some government-funded programs, including TRICARE and the Veteran's Administration; Worker's Compensation; and some other programs.

DEFINITION:

"Total drug costs" is the total of all payments made for your covered Part D drugs. It includes:

- What the plan pays.
- What you pay.
- What others (programs or organizations) pay for your drugs.

Learn more. Medicare has made the rules about which types of payments count and do not count toward "out-of-pocket costs" and "total drug costs." The definitions on this page give you only the main rules. For details, including more about "covered Part D drugs," see the *Evidence of Coverage,* our benefits booklet (for more about the *Evidence of Coverage,* see Section 6).

Chapter 12

Dealing with Problems Under Medicare

Maria Sanchez was having difficulty understanding why she was getting a bill from her local hospital. She'd recently been to the emergency room for leg pain. They had made copies of her Medicare card and her Medigap Plan F card. She had purchased that plan specifically because she didn't want to have to worry about being covered in situations like this. Something seemed amiss, so she called the hospital billing office for an explanation. Lo and behold, when she told the person on the phone that she didn't think she should be receiving an extra bill, an "error" was found—she didn't owe anything at all.

Balance Billing

All providers that treat Original Medicare patients—whether participating or non-participating— agree to abide by Medicare's billing rules. As a result, the maximum amount such a provider can expect to be paid is based totally on Medicare's approved fees, not on the provider's regular fees. For physicians, this is either 100% of the Medicare-approved fee or 109.25% of it, depending on whether or not they participate. For other types of providers the calculations are different, but there remains a maximum that the provider can expect to receive from Medicare plus any Medigap coverage plus the patient. All providers of any kind who accept payments from Medicare must adhere to these rules.

⚠️ **Any attempt to bill for more than the maximum amount allowed by Medicare is called *balance billing*. It's a violation of federal law. If you think it's happened, immediately question the bill.**

Unfortunately, balance billing occurs quite commonly. A patient receives a bill stating what was charged and what was paid by Medicare plus Medigap and noting that the remainder is due from the patient. In fact, nothing is due since the entire Medicare-approved fee has been paid.

Such practices may be purposely deceitful or only clerical errors. They happen with enough frequency that it strains the imagination to believe they are all simply mistakes. Some patients, erroneously believing that the balance is really their responsibility, pay the bill and the provider gets a windfall. Those who question such bills are usually told that an error was made and the charges are immediately eliminated, just as in Maria's case. It's amazing how quickly charges of this type get removed when they're challenged!

⚠ **Don't be one of the unaware who pay bills they don't really owe. Before paying any bill, make sure you're not being charged more than the Medicare-approved fee for a participating provider or the limiting fee for a non-participating one. Question any bill you don't understand.**

Questioning a Bill

Bills that you receive from all sorts of providers, but especially hospitals, can be extremely confusing. There can be many line item charges, each with an elaborate billing code but no written explanation of what service was really provided. How can you possibly understand a bill containing only codes? You can't. Theoretically, if you have Original Medicare and a Medigap Plan F, you should never get a bill from a hospital or any other provider, since all the charges should be 100% covered. That's why I like that plan so much. With any other Medigap plan, you may have to sort through a very long list of separate charges and check every one. Always reconcile such charges against the Medicare Summary Notice (Medicare's EOB) you get in the mail or against your claims data on the MyMedicare.gov website, as well as your Medigap plan's EOB.

If you believe a bill that you've received is not correct or if you simply don't understand it, the first thing you should do is call the provider or billing service. There should be a telephone number somewhere on the bill. Make sure you have the following in front of you when you call:

1. The actual bill that you are questioning.

2. Your Medicare Summary Notice, which includes the dates of service that are covered by the bill, or the EOB from your Medicare Advantage carrier (or comparable information from the appropriate website).

3. If you have a Medigap Plan, the EOB from the insurance company for the same dates.

4. A list of what you believe to be the services you received from the provider, including dates. Hopefully you have kept a detailed record of all medical services you received. If you haven't, try to reconstruct as best you can exactly what was done and when.

If you feel comfortable calling the provider/billing service on your own, great, but many people prefer to have another person who is more knowledgeable about medical billing help them. This might be your spouse, your child, or a volunteer at a senior center. However, you cannot simply ask someone else to call for you, since the provider/ billing service will almost assuredly refuse to talk to anyone but you. Strict federal laws regarding privacy of medical information (called *HIPAA regulations*) prevent them from dealing with anyone but you unless you specifically grant them permission to speak with someone else.

The simplest way to deal with this problem is for both you and the person helping you to be on the phone when you call. You will say something like "Hello. My name is _____ and I'm calling about my bill. My account number is _____ [It will be on the bill]. Also on the phone is my daughter, Sarah Green. I authorize her to talk to you on my behalf." The representative will probably verify who you are and your wishes regarding your daughter. From that point on, your daughter can do all the talking for you.

You may or may not be happy with the information you get. Sometimes a simple clarification is all that's needed. On occasion, the representative will find that an error was, in fact, made and will fix the problem. If you feel that you haven't gotten an adequate explanation, request additional information. Many times a bill will indicate only a range of dates of service and a total amount due. Ask for a *complete accounting* of all the services rendered.

For every service, this should show what was done, the date, the fee, how much was allowed by Medicare and paid by Medicare, how much was paid by a Medigap policy (if applicable), and any balance due from you. This should be sent to you, usually by mail. If they require a written request, send it right away. Make sure to keep a copy. Once you've reviewed the detailed accounting, call them back if you still have questions. For you to be satisfied, the representative must be able to explain exactly what you're being billed for and why you still owe money. Make sure you *always* get the name of the person you talked to on the phone.

If you still believe something is amiss—either you are being billed for services you didn't receive or all the services should have been paid for by Medicare and a Medigap policy (i.e., that you're being balance-billed)—your next call should be to Medicare at 1-800-MEDICARE. This should be your last call, not your first one. Always give the provider—whether doctor, hospital, laboratory, or durable goods supplier—the opportunity to explain or rectify the problem. Calling Medicare will result in an investigation. That may well be justified. Just make sure that you've exhausted other avenues before making that call.

Why not simply call Medicare first?

1. If you don't believe that the provider has given you an acceptable explanation or remedied the problem reasonably, you can always contact Medicare later. There's no deadline.

2. You should be aware that reporting a physician to Medicare is a very big deal for him. It will initiate an investigation that will create work for the office manager and aggravation for the physician. An honest doctor will be very troubled that his integrity is being questioned. You certainly have the right to contact Medicare, but make sure you understand the implications of doing so. Assuming that the problem was, in fact, only a clerical error, how do you think the doctor will feel toward you? Do you think you'll get the same care and empathy from him in the future? You won't. If you want to maintain the patient-doctor relationship, you would be wise to think twice before filing an official complaint without first checking with the doctor's staff.

Appeals

As you utilize your Medicare benefits, situations may arise in which you disagree with a decision made by a hospital, a skilled nursing facility, the contractor that administers Original Medicare in your area, your

Medicare Advantage plan, or your Medicare Drug Plan. You may feel that the ruling was made using faulty information or reasoning, or simply that the decision was unfair or unjust. In such situations, you have the right to appeal.

Earlier we talked about your rights if you believe you are being discharged from a hospital too soon or you have been informed that you no longer meet Medicare's criteria for continued coverage in a skilled nursing facility. In these cases, you may request a ruling from an independent outside organization contracted by Medicare. At the time a hospital or SNF informs you of its decision, you should be supplied with written information regarding how to appeal. If not, ask for it.

You may also appeal if a Medicare Advantage plan or a Medicare Drug Plan denies your request for a specific service, supply, or prescription drug that you feel you are entitled to. You might be requesting preapproval or seeking reimbursement for something you already paid for. Some examples include:

- Your PCP requests approval for a certain type of scan to help diagnose your problem, but your Medicare Advantage plan denies it.

- Surgery has been recommended by your PCP, but your Medicare Advantage plan won't approve the specific procedure that your surgeon suggests.

- Your doctor feels you need a specific medication, but that particular drug is not on your drug plan's formulary. The plan denies your request that it pay for that drug, noting that there are alternatives on the formulary.

Since Original Medicare generally does not require preapprovals, most appeals result from payment denials by the Medicare contractor after the fact. For whatever reason, a service has been deemed not medically necessary or inappropriate, or it was performed sooner than allowed (for example, routine colonoscopies are permitted only every 10 years). The physician or other provider receives the denial from Medicare and informs you that you are responsible for the bill; alternatively, you may see the denial when checking the MyMedicare.gov website or when you receive your Medicare Summary Notice in the mail (which now includes a form for filing an appeal entitled "How to Handle Denied Claims or File an Appeal").

Note that nothing has been mentioned about Medigap denials. Remember, all Medigap policies must pay when Medicare pays. The only possible cause for an appeal would involve a Medigap carrier contending that a service fell under a pre-existing condition exclusion.

For all of these situations, appeals processes are available to you. The details regarding how to file each type of appeal are complicated and unique to each situation. Medicare provides a brochure entitled *Medicare Appeals,* which is available from Medicare in printed form or as a downloadable pdf file at www.Medicare.gov/Pubs/pdf/11525. pdf. There's also information on the Medicare.gov website. (At the top of the home page, click on the sixth tab from the left, entitled *Claims and Appeals.*) For appeals of decision by Medicare Advantage plans or Medicare Drug Plans, the plan documents (which you received from the plan when you initially enrolled and should continue to receive yearly) will contain a detailed explanation of the appeals process—typically about 50 pages in length.

In all cases, there are five levels of appeal available to you:

- **Level 1**—Original Medicare: For claims that were denied, the initial step is redetermination by the Medicare contractor that handled the claim. If the appeal deals with your feeling that a hospitalization, skilled nursing facility stay, or home health service is being terminated too soon, then the determination is made by a Quality Improvement Organization (QIO).

  Medicare Advantage plans and Medicare Drug Plans: Reconsideration of the request is initially done by the plan.

- **Level 2**—Review by an outside organization. For Original Medicare, this is called a *Qualified Independent Contactor;* for Medicare Advantage plans and Medicare Drug Plans, it's an *Independent Review Entity.*

- **Level 3**—A hearing before an *Administrative Law Judge.*

- **Level 4**—Review by the *Medicare Appeals Council.*

- **Level 5**—Review by a *Federal District Court.*

During this process, you will need to provide documentation from your physicians and other providers to bolster your case. You are entitled to representation, including an attorney, but the costs must be borne by you. Some patient advocacy groups can provide assistance. One such organization is the Center for Medicare Advocacy, Inc., which has offices in Connecticut and Washington, DC. Its website is www. medicareadvocacy.org ; telephone number is 1-800-262-4414.

Most Level 1 appeals take one to several weeks. However, in some situations you are entitled to what's called a *fast appeal*—when delay could potentially be harmful to you. Sometimes fast appeals are automatic, such as review by a QIO regarding hospital discharge or stopping SNF treatment. This type of rapid determination applies equally to Original Medicare and Medicare Advantage plans. If you are requesting a medication not normally covered by your Medicare Drug Plan and your physician feels immediate use of the medication is critical, you can similarly request a *fast decision* and later a *fast appeal* if an initial request is denied.

⚠ **If you are contemplating any request for a preapproval or an exception, or considering any type of appeal, I strongly suggest you read the publication *Medicare Appeals* before doing anything else.**

Fraud and Abuse

There is absolutely no question that Medicare fraud is a huge problem. Estimates of the cost to Medicare of fraudulent claims vary greatly, partly because some studies include Medicare and Medicaid together. However, a number in the area of $50 billion per year is talked about. Whatever the exact figure, it represents a significant loss to Medicare at a time when the program is becoming costlier every year and calls for cuts in Medicare spending are getting louder. You might ask, "Why should Medicare fraud be important to me?" The answer is simple. The more money that is extracted from the system by fraud and abuse, the less will be available to pay for legitimate medical needs.

Much of the fraudulent behavior is perpetrated by large entities that systematically cheat Medicare (and Medicaid). They might bill Medicare for services never provided to hundreds or thousands of individuals under their care or bill for services to recipients they don't treat at all but whose Medicare numbers have been stolen. These large, obviously egregious practices are being investigated by CMS, but the process can be arduous. Part of the problem involves the fact that Medicare pays claims when they are submitted and only checks for fraud afterward. The money is already gone by the time an audit or investigation discovers the fraud. The perpetrators may ultimately be prosecuted, but little money recovered. It would obviously be preferable if fraudulently billed claims could be intercepted and payment withheld, but that is difficult since CMS attempts to pay claims (the vast majority of which are legitimate) rapidly. CMS has started to employ a new Fraud Prevention System to screen claims in an attempt to identify those that have suspicious characteristics before they are paid. As this system matures, it will hopefully help substantially.

All fraud is not the sole province of large organizations. It can be done in an almost endless variety of ways by doctors, nurses, clinics, home health agencies, durable goods suppliers, and inpatient institutions of all types. Here are but a few examples.

- A doctor performs a test or procedure that wasn't really needed.

- A nurse sends a patient to a particular lab or X-ray facility and gets a kickback for doing so.

- A hospital admits patients from the ER when they didn't really require hospitalization.

- A durable goods provider supplies a product of inferior quality and bills Medicare for a better one.

- A physician certifies that a patient qualifies for home care when she really doesn't, and the home care agency remunerates him.

- A nursing facility falsifies how much therapy a patient really received.

- A doctor upgrades the coding for an office visit beyond what is justified by the amount of work done.

Unfortunately the list is endless. What can you do to help? Here are a few suggestions:

- Always check your EOBs. If you see anything that doesn't look right, don't pass it by. As mentioned earlier, when it's from a provider you definitely used, first call the billing office with questions. When the provider is unknown to you, especially when the type of service, the date of service, or the location is preposterous, consider contacting Medicare right away.

- Never give your Medicare number to anyone other than a provider you have chosen to see. When you go to a doctor's office, a laboratory, or the hospital, they'll obviously need your Medicare number. *No one else needs it or is entitled to it.* Never give it to someone who calls you offering any kind of service and telling you that all you have to do is provide your Medicare number and it will be free. Such solicitations are virtually always fraudulent. They're stealing your Medicare number.

- Check out Medicare's excellent website regarding Medicare fraud. You'll find it at: http://www.stopmedicarefraud.gov. There's a tremendous amount of information there, including a box you can click to report fraud directly. The appropriate telephone numbers are there as well. For those who don't like using the Internet, the numbers are:

  ➤ Office of the Inspector General, U.S. Department of Health and Human Services: 1-800-HHS-TIPS (1-800-447-8477)

  ➤ Medicare itself: 1-800-MEDICARE (1-800-633-4227)

Chapter 13

The Future of Medicare

"I'm scared and angry," thought Warren Evans. "I've worked hard my whole life. I paid all my taxes—income tax, FICA, Medicare. Now that I'm 67 and getting all these health problems, the politicians are talking about getting rid of Medicare. If I hadn't gotten that nuclear stress test that showed my heart blockages, I might be dead. And what if I hadn't seen the dermatologist who found my skin cancer? Or had that colonoscopy where they got rid of the polyp? Sure, they say that people on Medicare now won't be affected. I don't believe that for a second. They want to give me a voucher to buy private insurance? It was an insurance company that wouldn't allow me to have a stress test like the one that found my heart problem—wasn't 'til I got on Medicare that my doctor could order it. Whatever the politicians come up with, it's not going to be good for people like me."

The future of Medicare is far from clear. The program created in 1965 to guarantee health care for Americans 65 and older is under attack. The reason: cost. Medicare as it now exists has become so expensive that it is becoming viewed as a burden on the economy. And the price tag for Medicare is rising, as the cost of delivering medical care increases, the number of baby boomers eligible for Medicare grows, and people live longer. By 2030, one in five Americans will qualify for Medicare. As a result, Medicare has become a major target for politicians of various stripes.

Medicare Meets ObamaCare

At first glance, the Affordable Care Act of 2010 (ObamaCare) appears to have little impact on Medicare recipients. Most provisions of the act relate to insurance coverage for Americans who aren't eligible for Medicare. It establishes health insurance exchanges to provide a marketplace of insurance options, subsidizes premium costs for individuals and small businesses, and prevents preexisting conditions from influencing the ability to obtain medical coverage. The most apparent alteration to Medicare policies is a progressive phasing out of the donut hole from Medicare Drug Plans (to be eliminated by 2020). Additionally, the Act made changes to the formulas for paying Medicare Advantage plans, including quality-based bonuses and penalties for underperforming plans.

Unfortunately, the belief that ObamaCare will not have more profound effects on Medicare is an illusion. In actuality, ObamaCare takes large amounts of its funding from Medicare. Nick Tate, in his excellent bestseller *ObamaCare Survival Guide,* has analyzed the impact of Obamacare on Medicare and concluded,

> Given the ocean of money funding Medicare it was inevitable that the authors of ObamaCare would tap into it to pay for the new health care system. As a consequence, senior citizens suffer the biggest financial blow from the new law. That's because Medicare's budget is cut by about $45 billion per year on average over the next ten years.[5]

The creators of ObamaCare have contended that much of the lost Medicare funding will be replaced by savings from reduced Medicare fraud, but it remains to be seen how effective the new antifraud efforts will prove to be. It is difficult to believe that $45 billion (with a "b") per year can be made up in this way.

The availability of care for seniors could easily be impacted as well. Tate further points out,

> About one-fifth of the funding for Obamacare (or $196 billion) will come from cuts to Medicare's payment rates to providers other than physicians over the next ten years.[6]

Hospitals, nursing facilities, and home health agencies will be the main targets of these cuts. As we have discussed earlier, insufficient Medicare reimbursement rates have resulted in many physicians limiting their Medicare practices or refusing to see Medicare patients at all. Nonphysician health care providers could take the same approach should Medicare fees drop low enough.

---

[5] Tate, Nick J, ObamaCare Survival Guide, Humanix Books, 2012 p.137

[6] Ibid., p. 142

Reductions in the amounts paid to Medicare Advantage plans have already begun. The likely results will be higher premiums and greater cost sharing for MA plan enrollees. Alternatively, insurance companies could simply depart the Medicare Advantage marketplace, leaving seniors with fewer (probably more expensive) options.

Critics of ObamaCare contend that cutting funding for Medicare to pay for ObamaCare is conscious social engineering intended to transfer health care from seniors to the poor, while ObamaCare supporters contend that cost savings from reducing waste will offset these cuts. Whatever the underlying motivation, it appears that under ObamaCare there will be fewer dollars to go around and greater constraints on Medicare services.

What Might the Future Bring?

The effects of ObamaCare and the strain that Medicare's costs are placing on the federal budget must inevitably result in substantial changes to Medicare. The question at hand is no longer whether federal outlays for Medicare will be controlled, but rather how limiting such expenditures should best be accomplished. Should Medicare recipients pay more for their coverage, as either higher premiums or greater cost sharing? Should benefits be curtailed? Should new models of delivering health care be incorporated? Or should the entire government-run system be junked and replaced by private insurance vouchers? Opinions vary greatly, based largely on sociopolitical and philosophical views. Proposed "fixes" are infrequently based solely on scientific and economic grounds.

What methods, then, are being considered to reduce Medicare's perceived burden on the economy? The one cost-containment measure that Medicare has already employed is limiting the amounts that providers of all types are paid for their services. Hospitals and physicians alike have seen little or no increases in their reimbursements for years; in many cases payment decreases have occurred. Further lowering the fees paid to physicians is unlikely, and reductions to other providers will be inadequate to produce significant additional savings. Other, more drastic means are being debated. Here is a listing of some of the changes you will see proposed for future versions of Medicare.

- **Increase the age of Medicare eligibility.** Changing the age for starting Medicare to 66 or 67, probably in increments of a few

months at a time, would result in fewer Medicare enrollees
and lower costs. Proponents argue that age 65 might have been
appropriate when Medicare was first conceived, but longevity
is so much greater now that benefits should start later. On the
other hand, many people have been waiting a long time to begin
Medicare so they can finally get adequate health coverage.
The effects of ObamaCare on this are unclear. With a higher
eligibility age, Medicare costs might be lower, while other
government programs might spend more subsidizing health
insurance for 65- and 66-year-olds.

- **Increase the premiums for more affluent Medicare recipients.**
  As previously discussed, higher premiums for Medicare Parts
  B and D presently apply to about 5% of recipients, based on
  modified adjusted gross income (MAGI). Premiums could be
  further increased for the 5%, or individuals with somewhat
  lower MAGIs could be charged extra premiums as well.

- **Change the regulations regarding Medicare Supplement
  Insurance plans (Medigap plans) to eliminate full coverage.** A
  plan that covers 100% of costs, the argument goes, promotes
  overutilization, since there are no financial incentives to avoid
  potentially excessive care. Proposals to change, eliminate, or tax
  Medigap plans are already on the table. Presumably Medigap
  plans could become less expensive, since they would provide
  less coverage.

- **Combine Medicare Parts A and B into one unified plan with
  a coordinated cost sharing structure.** The need for Medigap
  policies might be eliminated, or the structure of such plans
  altered significantly to preclude total coverage.

- **Curtail Medicare fraud.** Everyone agrees with this, but how
  much will be saved is unclear. The Affordable Care Act already
  has provisions to strengthen the federal government's ability
  to detect, prosecute, and hopefully deter Medicare fraud. More
  sophisticated methodology and greater enforcement powers
  created by the act have already helped. As these become more
  widely used, savings could potentially be significant. Not
  only could fraudulent billing be short-circuited before the
  claims were paid, but greater scrutiny and prosecution could
  discourage continued fraud.

- **Pay less for medicines.** The 2003 legislation that established Medicare Part D drug plans was weakened by a provision that prohibits Medicare from negotiating drug prices and benefiting from discounts like those received by other large drug purchasers. As a result, Medicare overpays for drugs, especially those administered in hospitals and in outpatient settings (such as intravenous chemotherapy). Intensive lobbying by the pharmaceutical industry and support from its friends in Congress were responsible for this. It could be changed with appropriate political will.

- **Establish which medical tests and interventions really work and which do not; then eliminate funding for those shown to be ineffective.** Some procedures and tests may be appropriate for certain patients, but inappropriate or wasteful for others. Only in recent years has the "appropriateness" of various procedures begun to be studied—the goal being to establish criteria for when specific interventions should (and should not) be done in various clinical scenarios. Careful examination of the effectiveness, safety, appropriateness, and risk-benefit ratios of procedures must be performed and the results implemented. Doesn't this make perfect sense? With funds so limited, why should Medicare pay for operations or medications that don't help or are less efficacious than others? And why should patients undergo procedures or tests, all of which have possible side effects, if they are of little value? Yet this apparently obvious concept has met with strident political opposition.

The Affordable Care Act created the Independent Payment Advisory Board (IPAB), a panel of 15 experts from various fields charged with reducing Medicare's costs, but specifically forbidden from rationing care. The board would make decisions without control by either the president or Congress, giving it great powers and theoretically protecting it from political pressure. Accused of interfering with decision making by doctors and patients, the IPAB has proven to be one of the most contentious elements of the Affordable Care Act. The board's effectiveness remains to be seen. Whatever the future of this controversial panel, means must be developed to control the use of wasteful, often expensive medical interventions of questionable value.

- **Control "defensive medicine" by changing the way in which medical malpractice claims are handled.** Everyone in medicine knows that doctors order many more tests than are needed. Physicians are fearful that if they don't order every conceivable study, some day they could be faulted in court. Trial lawyers contend that patients need to be protected from incompetent practitioners and compensated for their pain and suffering. However, physicians must be protected from liability if they follow "best practices guidelines" and utilize "evidence-based medicine" in their decision-making. Ordering every possible test and then repeating it "just to be sure" should not be required simply to avoid a liability suit. Tort reform must be a part of the overall approach to cost containment. We cannot justify reducing medical services for everyone, while at the same time keeping intact the ability of the few (and their attorneys) to receive large settlements.

- **Pay for medical care based on results, not services.** This involves an entirely different conceptual approach to medical care. CMS would contract with an organization that includes physicians, hospitals and other health care professionals to provide total care for a specific group of Medicare enrollees. You may hear about **Accountable Care Organizations (ACOs)**, which are models for delivering care in this manner. Pilot programs are beginning to appear around the country. Remuneration can be based on a fee-for-service model or on capitation, but in either case emphasis is placed on improving quality of care and cost containment. Control of utilization becomes the responsibility of the organization, and savings to Medicare can result in additional compensation for the ACO and its members.

- **Eliminate Original Medicare as it now exists and substitute a voucher system.** Each Medicare recipient would be given a specific amount of money (a voucher) to purchase private insurance. This is the type of fundamental change in the Medicare system that has been advocated by Rep. Paul Ryan, Gov. Mitt Romney's vice-presidential running mate in 2012. Costs would be contained, the argument goes, by competition in the insurance marketplace. Waste and inefficiency would be minimized by the various insurance companies having to compete for enrollees.

The obvious appeal of this plan is that the total federal outlay for Medicare would be known and predictable. Simply multiply the number of Medicare recipients by the amount that Congress authorizes per person and you've got the total cost. But how would the per-capita dollar amount be determined? What would happen, opponents ask, if the amount authorized by Congress was insufficient for the average senior to buy a meaningful policy? How much extra would each recipient have to pay out-of-pocket to get insurance? If the voucher amounts were too low, would people simply avoid buying anything? Or would they be forced to tolerate insurance that didn't provide for their needs? The insurance companies selling the policies would be making a profit. Couldn't this amount be better used paying for medical care?

- **Create a hybrid plan.** This is a variant of the voucher system. Each enrollee could use his voucher either to buy a private insurance policy or to pay for participation in some version of Original Medicare. This would allow for competition among plans, but still permit the survival of federally run Medicare. When you think about it, this is not unlike the present system, in which a senior can choose Original Medicare or a privately sponsored Medicare Advantage plan. This difference is how the private plans are funded. Under the present system, CMS pays the Medicare Advantage insurance carriers a per-capita amount based on the average cost of covering enrollees in Original Medicare. Under a voucher system, the dollar amount available to purchase private insurance or government-run Medicare would be predetermined by Congress.

Having finished this book, you should now be well versed in today's Medicare options—how to select them wisely and use them effectively. As the years go on, you will see many changes in Medicare—in how it's funded, in what it covers, in the choices you must make, and in the ways you'll access care. Medicare will no doubt continue to exist, but possibly in a very different form. Keep abreast of those changes and understand what they mean to you so you can continue to make the best decisions when choosing how you receive your medical care.

Appendix A

Original Medicare Preventive Care Examinations

Until fairly recently, Original Medicare's benefits specifically excluded preventive care. Annual routine physical exams and screening blood tests were not covered. Every examination or laboratory test was required to have a specific diagnosis attached to it and a specific reason it was being performed. Now, however, CMS has changed its policy to include and even emphasize preventive care, including a "Welcome to Medicare" exam during your first year of Medicare coverage and annual "Wellness" exams thereafter. Such exams are 100% covered by Original Medicare—i.e., there is no cost sharing.

Although Medicare emphasizes the importance of these exams for planning your subsequent health care, you should be aware that they are very definitely NOT complete physical exams. Here's what a "Welcome to Medicare" exam includes:

1. A review of your medical and social history including risk factors.

2. Measurement of your height, weight, blood pressure, visual acuity, and body mass index.

3. Education, counseling, and referrals.

4. A brief written plan for getting appropriate screening tests.

A doctor does not even have to touch you to provide this type of exam. She doesn't look into your mouth or ears, palpate your neck for lymph node or thyroid abnormalities, listen to your heart or lungs, feel your abdomen, check the strength of your pulses, or do any type of neurological testing. For women, there's no breast exam and certainly no internal exam. There's no rectal exam for either sex. In short, those of you who have had physical exams in the past will detect no similarity to what Medicare calls preventive health exams. In fact, a physician is not really needed to perform such an exam. All the elements listed under item 2. above are done by a medical assistant.

Certainly, the value of complete physical exams has been debated in medical circles. Some authorities feel they are not cost effective, stating that such exams yield little and take a lot of time. On the other hand, it's difficult to believe that eliminating virtually all elements of a traditional physical exam won't result in significant findings being missed. For example, a breast exam is an important addition to mammography in detecting breast cancer, since some breast lumps don't show up on routine mammograms. Similarly, a rectal examination to feel for prostate nodules is the best way to detect prostate cancer.

You should discuss with your doctor what elements of a true physical exam might be important to you and how they can be included in your plan of care.

Appendix B

Using the Medicare Plan Finder to Evaluate Medicare Part D Drug Plans

In order to use the Medicare Plan Finder to evaluate the various Medicare Drug Plan options available to you, go to www.medicare.gov and follow these directions. You will need a complete list of all your medications, including the dosages and how often you take them. The list needs to be precise. With that in hand, let's go through the following steps:

1. Once you've arrived at www.medicare.gov, which is the Medicare home page, click on the green button (near the top) entitled **Find health & drug plans.**

2. The next page will say *Medicare Plan Finder*. Enter your zip code in the box and click **Find Plans**.

3. *Step 1 of 4: Enter Information*. For the first question, click the appropriate information for you. I'd suggest clicking "Original Medicare," but you can also click "I don't have any Medicare coverage yet." For the second question, click the appropriate circle, which for most people will be "I don't get any Extra Help." Then click **Continue to Plan Results.**

4. *Step 2 of 4: Enter Your Drugs*. You will now enter each of the medications you presently take or will be taking in the near future. Make sure you know the dosage of each pill (usually in milligrams, abbreviated *mg* or *MG*) and how many you take. For each medication, the program will ask you the name, dosage, quantity, and frequency. Use the quantity you take in one month. Enter the drugs sequentially and the program will create an exact list. When you enter a drug's brand name, the program may tell you there's a generic available. Select whether or not you want the generic. Also, you will sometimes be asked to select a drug from a list, which may include your drug by itself, your drug in combination with other drugs, and sometimes even unrelated drugs that have similar names. Note that generic

drugs sometimes have a first name and last name. (For example, a common generic blood pressure medication called amlodipine is really amlodipine besylate.) The correct full name will be on your prescription bottle. Brand-name drugs virtually always have only a single name, such as Lipitor. When you've entered all your medications, click **My Drug List is Complete**.

5. Page *Step 3 of 4: Select Your Pharmacies*. On this page you can select up to two local pharmacies. Note that above the pharmacy list you are asked to select the number of miles the pharmacies may be from your zip code. It automatically uses one mile. Unless you're in a city, this number is too small. Select 6, 8, or 9—more pharmacies will appear. Pick two of them that you're likely to use, but *not* from the same pharmacy chain. Note that you may have more than one page of pharmacies to choose from (you'll see the number of pages at the lower left). Check **Continue to Plan Results**.

6. *Step 4 of 4: Refine Your Results*. Up to now, the questions have been straightforward. Now it gets trickier, since you'll have to make some choices.

   ➢ On the right side of the page, you'll see *Your Current Plan* if you selected Original Medicare in *Step 1*, or *Summary of Search Results* if you indicated you didn't have a plan in *Step 1*. There will be three choices here.

   ➢ Click the upper box that says **Prescription Drug Plans (with Original Medicare)**. The other two choices pertain to Medicare Health Plans (which are the same as Medicare Advantage plans). For now, don't click either of these two.

   ➢ On the left side of the page, it says **Refine Your Search**. Here you can click on boxes that will allow you to do things like specify premium limits or deductibles. I would suggest you *not* click on most of these until you have run through the program at least once. If you do, it will limit the number of plans that you will get to examine. It's best to see the maximum number of available options first. Later you can go back and enter refinements and see what happens to the results.

> ➢ <u>One exception</u>: Click the [+] at *Select Drug Options* (the 3rd button down). Four options will appear. Click the last box next to "provide mail order pricing" and then **Update Plan Results** at the bottom of the column.   Doing this will give you some useful information about mail ordering medications, which is usually more economical. It will not eliminate any plan choices.

> ➢ Finally, click **Continue to Plan Results** in the middle of the page.

7. You will now see ***Your Plan Results***. There will be information on quite a number of plans, created from the data you entered. The top box may be called **Original Medicare**. Don't be confused by this. It refers to drug costs if you have only Medicare Parts A & B but no Medicare Part D at all. It's useful only in that it illustrates how much you will be saving by having a Part D plan. Under **Prescription Drug Plans**, the program will tell you how many Medicare Part D plans match your preferences and will ask you how many you want to have displayed. Pick a large number so you can review lots of plans. Below that, it says **Sort Results By**. Click on the downward arrow and there will be a list of different criteria you can use to rank order plans. You can try different ones. I'd start with "Lowest Estimated Annual Retail Drug Cost." Click **Sort**.

8. Each Medicare Part D plan will appear in a large box. You'll see the plan name and the company that sponsors it. Below that will be detailed information about costs (using your specific drug list). You'll undoubtedly be most interested in the first column called **Estimated Annual Drug Costs**. These costs include the sum of all relevant premiums, deductibles, copays, coinsurance, and out-of-pocket cost in the donut hole. In comparing different plans, you'll immediately see that there may be huge differences in the annual costs.

> ➢ Look at column 4, entitled **Drug Coverage, Drug Restrictions, and Other Programs**. Pay particular attention to where it says **All Your Drugs Covered on Formulary**. For plans where it says Yes, the annual cost in column 1 will probably be lower than for plans where it says No. This makes sense, since your costs will be less when all your medications are on a plan's formulary.

> ➢ Also take particular note of column 5, where the Star Rating is shown. The Star Rating is a Medicare-created measure that includes data on member satisfaction, complaints, and handling of appeals. A rating of at least 3 (preferably 3.5) is desirable.

> ➢ You'll note that throughout the table you'll see the following sign: [?]. Click on any of them and you'll l see a definition or explanation of the term next to it. Try one.

9. Let's say you've looked at a number of the available plans and now you want to start refining your selection criteria. You can go back to the page called *Step 4 of 4: Refine Your Results* by clicking on **Return to Previous Page** (located at the top and bottom of the page). Once there, use the box on the left side of the page to refine your search. Suppose you want to limit your premium to no more that $40 per month. Click the [+] next to **Limit Your Monthly Premium** and you'll be able to slide the arrow back and forth to select a premium limit—in this case $40. Next you *must* go to the bottom of the column and click **Update Plan Results**. (If you omit this, it won't work.) After it processes, click **Continue To Plans Results** on the right side of the page and you'll get an updated plan list incorporating your new criterion. You can do this as many times as you want and can adjust as many criteria as you like.

Index

Page numbers where terms are defined are shown in **bold**.

U

Unethical acts, requesting of physician 138
Urgent Care Center (see Immediate Care Center)

V

Voucher system   208-209

W

Websites (see Internet sites)
Welcome to Medicare exam 41, 211-212
Wellness exam 41
Widow/widower 20
Wisconsin, special Medigap rules 55
Wound care center 164

About the Author

Ronald Kahan, MD, a sought-after health care lecturer and consultant, is an associate clinical professor at Yale School of Medicine and has practiced medicine for more than thirty years. He received his bachelor's degree from Yale University, his MD from Weill-Cornell Medical College, and went on to conduct his residency at Harvard combined hospitals, specializing in dermatology.

Born in 1945, Dr. Kahan is one of the millions of Americans now covered by Medicare. He has tackled Medicare issues in both his personal and professional life, which brings an incredibly rich, practical perspective to his writing.